Hospitals and the health care revolution

L. H. W. Paine
Formerly House Governor and Secretary,
The Bethlem Royal and Maudsley Hospitals,
London, England

and

F. Siem Tjam
Division of Strengthening of Health Services,
World Health Organization,
Geneva, Switzerland

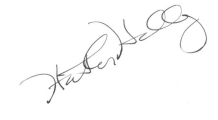

World Health Organization
Geneva
1988

TYPESET IN INDIA
PRINTED IN ENGLAND

87/7442—Macmillan/Clays—6000

Contents

He who has health
has hope, and he who has
hope has everything.

Arab proverb

Chapter 1. Symptoms of change

The fact that hospitals change is unremarkable. Whether they are in the wealthy industralized nations or the less well-off developing countries of the world, they are—or should be—dynamic institutions; and in any dynamic society the only constant is change. They are also, these days, to a greater or lesser extent depending on their circumstance and type, scientific and technological institutions; and as such they are subject to the rapid developments typical of modern-day science and technology.

But not all the changes that occur in hospitals are brought about by the discoveries of the scientists and the advances made by technologists. Some have economic roots and some stem from other aspects of man's unconquerable mind—from a desire for social equity, for example, a hatred of injustice, a wish to help the sick and disadvantaged, or a simple love of humanity.

It is with changes inspired by these latter beliefs that this opening chapter is concerned, changes that are naturally of local significance but may well be more important than that. For some of them give indications of what many now clearly see as a gradual but significant shift towards new ways of providing health care to the peoples of the world.

In short they are harbingers of something that is nothing less than a health care revolution. And the few precursory examples of this great event that we have chosen to present here have been deliberately titled as though they were the work of some eminent writer of what the libraries commonly call 'thrillers', because the trend they illustrate is indeed thrilling as well as a noble, humanitarian, and momentous one.

First, then, to the case of the disappearing walls.

The case of the disappearing walls

Hospitals in many countries today, either by design or by force of circumstance, are transferring clinical activities that were once undertaken only in the very heart of the institution—in wards, operating suites, and special units—to outpatient departments, day-care units, outreach programmes, and home and community care services. Many others show some interest in the promotion of health in the community through activities that are not necessarily based in the hospital.

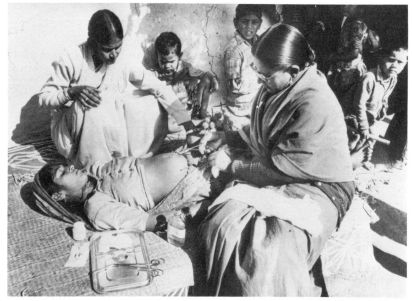

WHO Photo: J. Schytte

Many clinical activities are now being carried out in the community: here, a community health worker removes stitches from a wound.

Such actions are beginning to break through the carapace of assured self-containment with which many of the highly skilled, highly qualified professional staff of the hospital have too often surrounded themselves in the past.

2

All this means that those metaphorical hospital walls, no less real to the patients for being abstractions, are at last beginning to sway in the wind of change, and the day is surely coming, even though yet still some way off, when that wind will finally blow the walls to the ground.

Indeed, in a number of hospitals in various parts of the world, the constraining walls have largely disappeared as the institutions' traditional curative activities have been supplemented by many other functions, all intimately bound up with improving health but previously thought to be impracticable and of no direct concern to hospitals.

As an example of such an institution, none could be more appropriate than the Dr Carlos Luis Valverde Vega Hospital in San Ramón, Alajuela, Costa Rica.

This hospital introduced what it calls its 'hospital without walls' programme thirty years ago, and despite opposition and difficulties the programme continues today with remarkable achievements to its credit.

The philosophy of the experiment is best described in a paper written in 1985 by the hospital's Medical Director:

Successful health action is measured not just by what is done inside the hospital but, more importantly, by the initiatives taken within the hospital's area of influence. Consequently, it is the hospital's responsibility to carry health activities outside its own walls. This calls not only for proper dedication to curative and preventive medicine, but also for an understanding that the latter is above all a matter for the community, individually and collectively.

The hospital should also collaborate in activities aimed at improving the health and living standards of the population, by becoming involved in such matters as housing, land tenure, electricity supply, drinking water, roads, etc.

Resources and services should be distributed according to the needs of the community.

The ultimate aim is that the human being should live in the best conditions of individual, family and collective wellbeing.[1]

Working through, and with, five health centres, five social security clinics, and 46 health posts (which it helped to establish) distributed throughout the area, the hospital has been involved in raising living standards in the ways mentioned, in developing active community participation in

---

[1] GUIER, J.G.O. *Our first referral level hospital supported by the community and involved in primary health care within its catchment area through the "hospital without walls" experiment.* Unpublished WHO document, SHS/EC/85/WP/III.C.4.

the provision of health care, and in providing appropriate education and training for professional staff and community workers.

It has also been involved in a variety of other health activities ranging from regular weekend visits by its doctors and nurses to health posts in the remote parts of its area; similar regular visiting by interprofessional clinical teams to elderly chronic sick and disabled patients in the towns and villages around it; research and prevention programmes for hepatitis and tuberculosis; and improved treatment for those suffering from psychiatric and alcohol-related problems.

The paper provides statistical evidence of the improvements in the health of the people of Alajuela Province that have taken place in the last decade as a result of the 'hospital without walls' experiment, but as it points out, these indicators only partially reflect the aims and achievements of the programme.

> More important than these cold but significant figures is the experience accumulated by our communities in solving their problems jointly. This experience has become transformed into a social awareness which augurs well for future advances very soon.

Such advances are towards a vision of health that is far wider than that of most hospital staff today.

> Unfortunately the world's hospitals are measured in traditional terms, in the conventional care of the inpatient and out-patient. But they should seek to reach out beyond their walls, take part in the overall effort for comprehensive health care, and engage in bringing about changes both in the environment and in individuals within society.

And if this kind of advance is to be made in the foreseeable future it will require the full support of policitians, health care professionals, and people themselves.

> The hospital's role in primary health care should be coordinated and backed up by legislation, so that through decentralization of the health system with community participation, better living standards are attained more quickly. . .
> The sophisticated teaching hospitals should also become deeply involved in the teaching of this new approach to the hospital, for the traditional intra-mural attitudes are still creating difficulties for the development of programmes such as ours.

4

Dedicated concerted action by all interested parties will be necessary before the metaphorical walls of the world's hospitals are finally levelled.

But meanwhile let us look at another aspect of the evolving hospital scene—the way that the specialist services, of which the hospital is traditionally comprised, are themselves beginning to change.

The case of the disappearing specialists

It is appropriate to start this second of our three examples with an extract from another paper, written by another medical director, but this time about the Patan Hospital in Nepal.[1]

> Following the Alma-Ata Declaration[2] many hospitals were stimulated to develop primary health care activities outside the hospital walls. By contrast, when Patan Hospital was opened in November 1982, it was pledged to support an already existing and growing community primary health care programme in the Lalitpur District of Nepal. The reader is welcomed to enter the practical world of applying this policy, of facing the questions it raises and of formulating and attempting possible solutions to these questions.
>
> This is a world of trial, experience, and modification, of successes and failures. Satisfactory approaches at a given time and in a given situation may not work at another time or in another place.

The Patan Hospital is a fairly new institution. A district hospital of 140 beds, serving a mixed urban and rural population of 210 000, it is the product of joint planning by the Nepalese Government, the United Christian Mission (an international religious organization), and the local people. As indicated, it was opened in 1982 and is one of a number of general and specialist hospitals in the valley of Kathmandu, where 80% of the country's 690 doctors (1 per 25 000 people) work.

Nepal is one of the world's poorest countries with a per capita gross national product of approximately US $160 and a total population of just under 16 million in 1983. In such circumstances, its national health care plan may appear

---

[1] DICKENSON, J. G., *In support of primary health care: Patan Hospital, Nepal. A report.* Unpublished WHO document, SHS/EC/85/WP/III.C.1.

[2] See Chapter 2 and ref. 1.

somewhat ambitious, envisaging as it does that each of the country's 75 administrative districts should have a district hospital and 6–10 health posts manned by paramedical staff, each serving populations of 10–20 000, with this pattern of primary and secondary care further supported by a network of zonal, regional, and central hospitals.

Such a pattern does not necessarily require district hospitals of any great complexity. However, in many areas, such as the hilly terrain that makes up some two-thirds of the district served by Patan, there are no proper roads. A journey to the district hospital in Patan itself, therefore, from one of the most outlying villages, can involve one or two days on what the local people call 'the no 11 bus'—i.e., on foot.

Even, therefore, with more specialist hospitals available in nearby Kathmandu, the temptation must have been strong for the planners of the Patan Hospital to include facilities for medical and surgical subspecialities.

That this temptation was firmly resisted is much to their credit. The hospital was designed and built to meet four prime objectives—to provide primary health care services directly; to provide secondary care through departments of medicine, surgery, paediatrics, and obstetrics and gynaecology only; to support the local district community care services; and to help with national training programmes for health workers.

The result is that primary health care activities form a large part of the hospital's services both intra- and extramurally. Intrinsic to the design of the outpatient department is the concept of a 'health post within a hospital' manned by paramedical staff (health assistants and/or auxiliary nurse-midwives) and supervised by a family practitioner doctor, where the majority of self-referred patients are seen, diagnosed and treated.

The hospital also provides offices, meeting rooms, and educational facilities for the community primary health care services and, conversely, its doctors visit health posts in the district to gain experience and to support the local health workers.

Quite firmly and despite problems, the policy of the hospital is to provide care only at the primary and secondary levels, and to avoid developing tertiary or subspeciality services. In pursuing this innovative, courageous, and difficult path, the hospital is said to have been 'neither a shining success nor a total failure'. Problems remain, but are manifestly being tackled, and as an interesting facet of the case of the disappearing specialists, the experience in Patan represents a noteworthy signpost to the future.

Other such signposts undoubtedly exist in many countries, but we will content ourselves here with a brief mention of two more—the North Central Bronx Hospital in New York, USA, and the Ramathibodi Hospital in Bangkok, Thailand (2).

Among a number of creative ideas put into practice by the North Central Bronx Hospital in order to improve the health of the deprived people it serves, a Neighborhood Family Care Center was set up in 1973, oriented, as its name implies, towards treating families rather than disease. The general medical, paediatric and subspeciality clinics previously provided at the centre were phased out and replaced by five primary health care teams, each acting as an independent unit responsible for the comprehensive care of a particular group of families in the district. The teams are 26 to 28 strong and include junior doctors, nurse practitioners, social workers, community nurses, and family health technicians.

The Ramathibodi Hospital is a teaching hospital associated with the Mahidol University in Bangkok. It was opened in 1969 and has since developed a Community Health Programme and Department. The primary objectives of the teaching activities in community health are:

(a) To offer an integrated and progressive sequence of learning experiences which will give students the knowledge and skills needed for a critical examination of the health care needs of a defined population, and for the design of health care programmes to meet their needs.

(b) To prepare students and junior doctors to perform effectively as first-class health centre physicians, giving the best possible comprehensive and integrated health care—curative, preventive and promotive—to the people of the district using the limited resources available at such health centres.

7

As Dr R. Macagba says in his report on this development (2):

In summary the major goal of the community health programme is to develop in students the ability and motivation to think of health care not just in terms of doctors practising curative medicine with individual patients, but also in terms of community health care, which is defined as the provision of comprehensive, integrated health care (curative, preventive and promotive) to a defined population group by a team of health workers led by a physician. . . . It took the visit of consultants from abroad and attendance at international meetings to make some of the leaders in the hospital more aware and convinced of the importance of adjusting the medical care system to the needs of the people. Feedback from the graduates revealed that what was being taught in medical school was not relevant to the community. There was too much specialization in the hospital.

This brings us to the last of our selected examples of harbingers of the health care revolution—the case of the disappearing conventions—and here it is necessary to do no more than give a few illustrations of trends and practices that demonstrate how the traditional ideas on appropriate hospital and health care are changing.

The case of the disappearing conventions

The activities now undertaken by some hospitals must cause surprise, and perhaps concern, to the traditionalists.

We have already touched upon some of these activities in our comments on the 'hospital without walls' programme, and two others worthy of mention concern the Holy Family Hospital in Bihar, India, and the Gonoshasthaya Kendra, or Peoples' Health Centre Trust, in Bangladesh.

At the Holy Family Hospital, for example, one of the 14 departments is not a clinical one at all, but is a Farm Department run by a graduate of the College of Agriculture; in addition, the hospital's Community Health Department, set up in 1974, has a staff of eight, led not by a doctor or a nurse but by an agricultural worker. The team includes auxiliary nurse-midwives, an adult education worker, and a tractor driver! Retired administrators of large psychiatric hospitals, which once went in for large-scale farming as patient therapy, are probably among the few health professionals in the developed world today who will not find such activities strange.

The Gonoshasthaya Kendra integrates its small hospitals into a primary health care and rural community

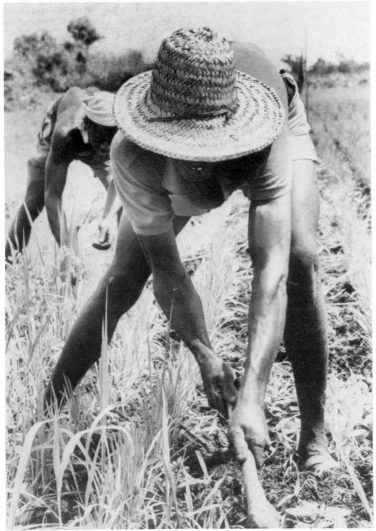

WHO Photo: E. Mandelmann

Agriculture and health—two closely related sectors.

development programme designed to improve the health of the poor people of Bangladesh. This programme is largely a non-hospital one and consists *inter alia* of agricultural extension groups, the promotion of education, training and

9

employment of women, and the cooperative commercial production of essential drugs.

Unusual perhaps, but highly appropriate to the local circumstances and firmly supported by the local population, you might think? But no! Among the obstacles and problems encountered in the development of this manifestly humane programme, has been the murder of workers for the Trust because 'health is a political issue and those enjoying care do not want to share it' (2).

Apart from such unusual innovations in developing countries, more obvious general trends have been observable for quite a few years which illustrate the considerable changes that are taking place, particularly in doctor–patient relationships and in the ways in which hospitals treat their customers.

Compulsory listing of the ingredients of drugs; explanatory health leaflets; consent forms for surgical procedures; patients' advocates; health service ombudsmen; non-negligence compensation schemes; medical malpractice insurance; quality assurance programmes; and the establishment, in Italy, of an international organization for the humanization of hospitals, all testify to the slow but steady decline of the 'lie still, do as you are told, keep quiet, and we'll make you better' school of paternalistic medicine.

It is a decline to which WHO has been looking forward for some time. Fifteen years ago, in a working party report to the Executive Board on promoting the development of basic health services (3), it was proposed that, in order to implement such a policy on a worldwide basis, there were three prerequisites. The first two, as might be expected, were "a health service structure capable of taking action" and "proper management". The third was not quite so obvious:

... the health services must really be accepted by the persons they serve. It is not difficult to understand why health services have developed as a system imposed upon populations—something that comes into a town or village from the outside. Medical literature and project proposals are filled with terms such as "acceptors", "refusal rates", "problem families", "under utilization", which show clearly that the problem is seen as a failure on the part of people, rather than as a failure of the health services. What is necessary now is to solicit community identification with, and participation in, the development of health services. This will require innovative approaches.

10

As Dr T. A. Lambo, Deputy Director-General of WHO, put it in his opening remarks to the meeting of the Expert Committee on the Role of Hospitals at the First Referral Level:

To increase the momentum of Health for All, to improve interaction between hospitals and other services in the community and to reorient hospitals to a local health system based on primary health care, questions should be asked on how the functions of the first-referral level can be better performed by local hospitals, whether they are small rural institutes or mammoth general hospitals in urban areas. Having recognized the limitations of the medical technology approach to Health for All we should move to identify new ways in which hospitals can contribute more effectively towards the social goals for health. We should avoid falling into the trap of "medicalization" of primary health care and bring our collective experience and wisdom to bear on clarifying the issues concerning hospitals at the first referral level.

Chapter 2. The health care revolution

The dictionary tells us that a revolution is a great upheaval or a complete change in, for example, outlook, social habits or circumstances. The world has known many such revolutions, some involving the sort of sudden and catastrophic change that the word implies, others being of longer duration and gentler effect. The health care revolution, as we understand it, is a great change of the more gradual kind. At its simplest, the health care revolution, as we implied in the previous chapter, is an attempt to integrate hospitals into a new style of health care system centred on primary health care.

More expansively, it could be described as an international crusade founded on the principle that health is a basic human entitlement, to which all should have equal access and an equal right, irrespective of nationality, residence, wealth or social position; for the achievement and maintenance of which all should take some responsibility, in relation to themselves and to others; and in the pursuit of which everyone must be concerned—with doctors and other professional health workers playing a major and essential role, but not necessarily the predominant one.

This last point—the part that medicine plays in the achievement of collective good health—is particularly relevant to an exposition of the health care revolution. For while doctors and other health professionals would probably accept that, despite their best efforts, the main determinants of good health remain largely outside their domain, what they are much less likely to agree to is that modern medical care, in practice, is not necessarily synonymous with good health care.

In their book *The struggle for health* (4), Sanders & Carver ask the pertinent question "Why is health care so inappropriate?" and then proceed to answer that question as follows:

> Both in the underdeveloped and in the developed world the medical contribution is largely inappropriate to health needs and does not cope with the health problems of the vast majority.
>
> The germ theory of disease and advances in medical science created the basis for what has been termed 'the bio-engineering approach' to illness. This approach persists today where a patient is regarded as a set of systems, one or more of which go wrong in illness, and which health workers attempt to put right with drugs and high technology. But most illness in the developed and underdeveloped world has its origins in social conditions.

The advent of the health care revolution is seen throughout the world—certainly in most Member States of WHO—as being directly linked, in many instances, to the inability, unwillingness or failure of established medicine to meet the health needs of the people.

The reasoning behind such a view has been expressed many times and in many ways by a variety of critics, but never more explicitly than in an article entitled "Health—a demystification of medical technology", which appeared in the *Lancet* as long ago as 1975 (5).

Here, under the subheading of "The mystery holders", is what the author, Dr Halfdan Mahler, Director-General of WHO, had to say about the contribution of the medical establishment to the health needs of the people. Although he refers directly to the health scene in Europe and North America, his arguments are universally applicable:

> The wave of social consciousness in the 19th century in Europe and in North America broadened our understanding of "Health" but resulted in a reaction by the medical Establishment and a constriction which is still continuing. By legislation, by training, by organisation, and by the way in which health-related interventions are stated and restricted, there has been a progressive "mystification" in medical care which is continuing almost unchecked. As our understanding of cause and effect has grown, "medicine" has continued to restrict the range of problems for which it considers itself responsible and the gap between "health care" and "medical care" has become ever wider. This has been coupled with an organisational change which has influenced the manner of dealing with these problems, a gross restriction in the information available and decisions to be made by people outside the health professions, and an unnecessary but inevitable dependency of the population upon the holders of these mysteries.
>
> If true, this is a grave charge. As with such general charges the evidence adds up to suspicion rather than certainty. If one looks back to the last century in England, the attack upon some of the physical evils of the Industrial Revolution was clearly led by social reformers, such as the

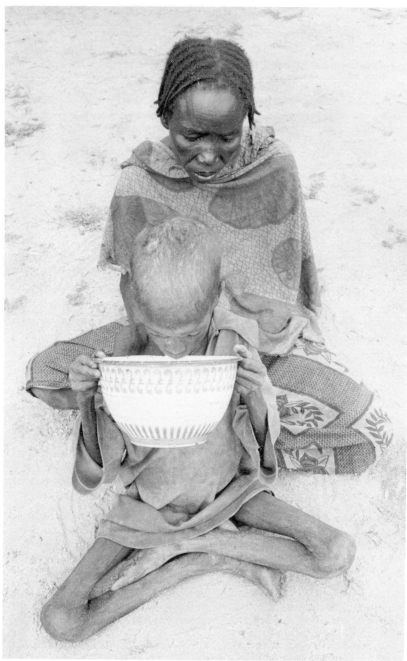

WHO Photo Competition: Liliane de Toledo

"Most illness . . . has its origins in social conditions".

Chadwicks, the health professions having secondary roles such as certifying most questionably the health effects of rising damp and back-to-back houses. There was a change in the disease picture (especially the communicable diseases) but the evidence linking this to medical improvement interventions rather than to changes in the society and the environment is also questionable. The continuing decreases in incidence and mortality appear to be largely extensions of continuing trends and were not directly related, in time, to immunisation or to direct medical action.

In parallel with these changes in disease pictures came a change in distribution of health resources. On the one hand there was the expansion of coverage to the universality of access which you now have, and on the other came the increased expenditure of specialised resources upon the few. This meant that a widening of the base did not result in a lowering of the peak or a flattening of the health expenditure pyramid. The peak is still rising higher, but this time it is a peak of expenditure directed towards the few, selected not so much by social class or wealth but by medical technology itself. Such an evolution is a world-wide rather than a peculiarly national trend. In some places where it has been examined it has been identified as an increasing expenditure upon persons in the final months or years before death. It appears that this expenditure does not measurably increase life expectancy or make humanly tolerable the closing episodes of the lives of elderly people. In other countries the increased expenditure on the few has been linked to the "upgrading" of health care interventions to higher and higher levels of the medical Establishment. This is typified by a statement of intent, within a developing country with a high maternal and neonatal mortality, that the medium-term objective will be to arrange that every woman in labour should be delivered by a consultant specialist obstetrician. Many other examples of the same trend can be cited. When added together they appear to say that health workers consider that the "best" health care is one where everything known to medicine is applied to every individual, by the highest trained medical scientist, in the most specialised institution. This type of thinking is clearly as dangerous as it would be for me, who spends so much time flying from Member State to Member State, if I preferred the aircraft in which I was travelling to be flown by a professor of aeronautical engineering rather than an experienced pilot.

If one follows this same line of thought one understands the inevitable side-effect that, as health care action moves higher and higher up the referral ladder, it comes to be justified more ·and more by the actions themselves and is more restricted. It is frightening but expected that when a specialised group is formed to perform certain actions it is evaluated and continues to be supported because of the *number* of such actions which it does, rather than by whether a problem is solved. There are counter-reactions to such trends well typified by the recent public debate over the treatment of spina bifida. Another example of reaction to this path could be a children's burn unit in a major city which showed that many of its intake of cases resulted from injuries caused by scalding coffee in the home. Rather than conducting research upon a more effective treatment of burns it directed its attention to the design of a coffee-pot which would not spill. The wide acceptance of the new design led to a decreased number of cases. But these exceptions make existing trends even more frightening.

Such trends towards restricted high technology might be said to be a byproduct of medical research distortions, and a good case might be made for directing a portion of the blame to the priorities of research-workers supported for the most part from national funds. But such finger-pointing

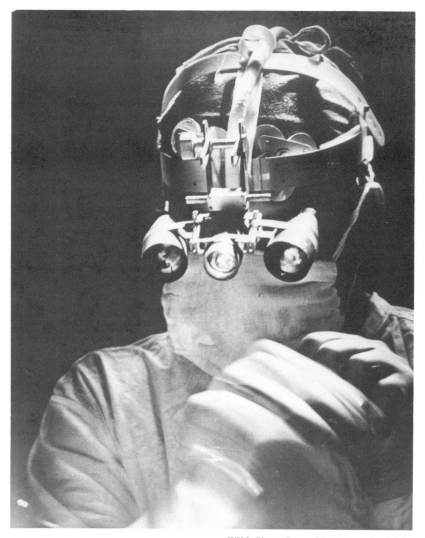

WHO Photo Competition: Alexander Ptitsin

"The mystery holders"

cannot explain all that is happening. The movements of interventions further up the professional ladder and the increased restriction of action to fewer and fewer people does not seem to be related only to new research findings. The implications of such a movement are not only seen as an increase in costs with few measurable health advantages in terms of either morbidity of mortality: they are also seen as a down-grading in social status of health workers at the bottom of the pyramid, changing aspirations of health workers who understandably want to be legitimised to as high a point in the pyramid

16

as possible, or public reaction such as the disturbances in the United States of America caused by the increase in malpractice litigation.

Dr Lambo, in his opening comments to the meeting of the WHO Expert Committee on the Role of Hospitals at the First Referral Level, said much the same thing in different words.

Over the past twenty years there has been increasing dissatisfaction about the relevance and effectiveness of national health systems in the developing as well as in industrialized countries. The highly sophisticated and very costly medical technologies usually concentrated in hospitals have been seriously questioned in the light of their social relevance and effectiveness for the health of people.

People became aware that physicians were not the only human resource to be used in all cases, hospitals were not the only way to provide health care, and the medical model was not the only possible foundation for a national health system.

As a result, the world community recognized that the alternative approach of primary health care involving the totality of all potential resources and based on equity and justice, individual and community self-reliance and intersectoral cooperation, including community involvement, would promote and achieve faster and more efficiently the goals of Health for All.

Until recently, a "central" notion dominated ideas concerning the role of hospitals in the health care system. The hospital was considered to be the centre, providing leadership and guidance to all other forms of health care, and the medical technology approach very much determined the shape of health systems.

But as is now becoming increasingly accepted, the hospital-centred health care system, while bringing many benefits to its users, does not of itself satisfactorily address the health needs of the people, especially those in developing countries, which do not necessarily have complementary social benefits such as satisfactory housing, employment, education, nutrition, clean water supplies, and efficient sewerage systems.

Hospitals, for understandable reasons, have for the most part developed as institutions isolated from the lives and comprehension of the mass of the people. This isolation has been, if anything, exacerbated by the march of modern scientific medicine over the past 50 years or more.

The gulf that has developed between these scientific temples of healing and the basic health requirements of the population, and the main reasons for the development of that gulf are well explained in a background paper on the role of hospitals in primary health care, prepared by WHO for a conference on this subject held in Karachi, Pakistan, in November 1981 (6).

In general, the hospital has developed as an enclosed building associated largely with curative activities performed for those individuals who find their way to the institution. In particular during the last half century or so, their development has not come about as a direct response to the major health needs and demands of the mass of the population in any particular country, or of the possibility of acting upon those needs and demands. The more sophisticated the hospital, the greater the cost implications and the wider the gap between [its] special capacities and the population's overall health needs and demands. This gap came to encompass the areas of teaching and research as well. Survey data from many countries show the limited catchment areas of so-called national referral centres. In Third World countries it is usual for 90 per cent of all in-patients in such institutions to be drawn from the city in which it is located. What are some of the major factors explaining the development of hospitals in the way described?

The paper continues by stressing the restricted ability of the poor to fulfil their needs for health care, for they are not in a position, economically or politically, to enjoy access to much health care of any kind—except possibly of the traditional type—and certainly not care based on costly high technology. Much formal health care planning aims at providing an overall coverage of the population with particular services (e.g., ensuring a certain number of doctors per 1000 population) and with sophisticated technologies, often in the absence of the proven relevance and benefit of the latter. This approach ignores not only the economic and political incapacity of the poor to purchase health care, but also the needs and priorities of the general public. It is here that community involvement can be of great importance in ensuring the relevance of health care services, through informed contributions to the development of health processes. Effective organization of the public can influence decision-making at all levels in favour of policies directed towards the achievement of health for all.

As has been stated, the modern hospital has not developed in response to the major health needs and demands of the mass of the population, and the possibility of positively acting upon those needs and demands. One basic reason, as discussed, has been the weakness of the poor: another has been the external influences brought to bear upon the hospital; external, that is, to mass health needs and demands. The major such external factor has been technology itself. Undoubtedly, many of the technological innovations of recent years have been positive in terms of the number of people who have benefitted from them. It is equally certain that many of these technological innovations have had only marginally beneficial effects, while others have had no effect at all, and some have had . . . negative ones.

The economic environment of current health care systems provides some incentives and few discouragements to the adoption of the latest technology. Beginning with the subsidization of research and development, governments and industry provide relatively unconstrained conditions for 'buyers' and 'users' of health technologies. This situation is further perpetuated by various pressures resulting, for instance, from marketing campaigns, high public expectations concerning specialized medical care, the prevailing professional image of quality medical care (in terms of medical 'centres of excellence'), and even competitive aspirations for prestige. All of these contribute to relative, or absolute, overinvestment in costly medical care facilities . . .

The modern medical school and its teaching hospital are the product of a symbiotic relationship with industry which has produced the scientific and technological base on which the teaching hospital now rests. This particular symbiotic relationship substitutes for one between the hospital and the whole population which would be based upon mass health needs and demands. The existing relationship between the hospital and the producers of high technology extends beyond the immediate uses of all possible available technologies, to the training of future medical practitioners, and to research efforts as well. Medical students are [usually] trained to pursue a 'technological imperative', to use any available technique of intervention— sometimes even in the absence of clearly proven effectiveness, regardless of cost, if there is any possibility at all of medical gain no matter how limited.

The problems connected with application of the 'technological imperative' are greatly exaggerated in conditions of sharp resource constraints. Thus, the external (to mass health needs and demands) technological factor is compounded in Third World countries by another factor external to them: that the latest technological innovations are developed by, and in the first place for use in the industrialized countries. The application of the technological imperative in countries spending annually as much US $1,000 per capita for health care creates sufficient havoc there, but when applied in countries spending one-tenth or one-hundredth or even one-thousandth of that amount for health care, the results are catastrophic!

So, as Dr Lambo went on to say in his address:

In the Primary Health Care philosophy and approach as embodied in the Declaration of Alma-Ata in 1978, the hospital came to be seen as part of a wider health system. Primary health care constitutes the foundation and the role of hospitals is to support it as referral and support mechanisms. The shift in perception has made many hospitals and professionals uneasy, but it provides, together with other socioeconomic imperatives, an impetus to both the public and private owner and operator to re-examine the position of hospitals with respect to primary health care.

The Declaration of the 1978 Conference at Alma-Ata in the USSR has been quoted many times but it is of such importance that it is worth reminding readers once again of the gist of what it said. The following is an extract from the Declaration (1).

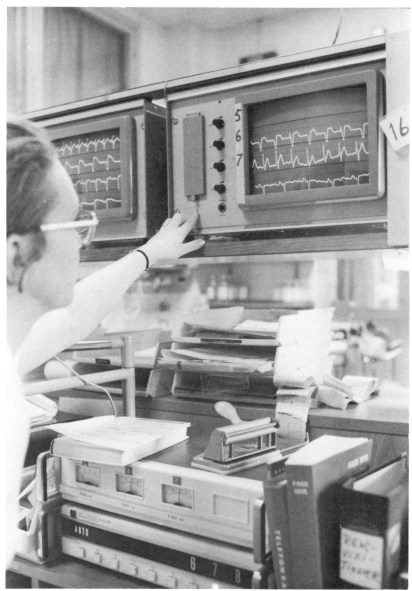

WHO Photo: E. Mandelmann

The "technological imperative".

Primary health care is essential health care based on practical, scientifically sound and socially acceptable methods and technology made universally accessible to individuals and families in the community through their full participation and at a cost that the community and country can afford to maintain in the spirit of self-reliance and self-determination. It forms an integral part both of the country's health system, of which it is the central function and main focus, and of the overall social and economic development of the community. It is the first level of contact of individuals, the family and community with the national health system, bringing health care as close as possible to where people live and work, and constitutes the first element of a continuing health care process.

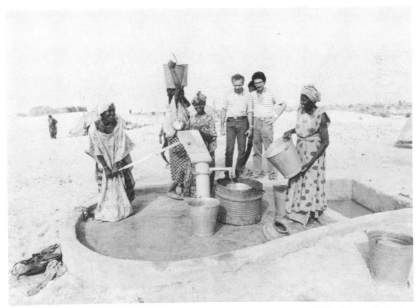

WHO Photo: B. Genier

A safe water supply makes a major contribution to health.

Primary health care:

1. reflects and evolves from the economic conditions and sociocultural and political characteristics of the country and its communities and is based on the application of the relevant results of social, biomedical and health services research and public health experience;
2. addresses the main health problems in the community, providing promotive, preventive, curative and rehabilitative services accordingly;
3. includes at least: education concerning prevailing health problems and the methods of preventing and controlling them; promotion of food supply and

21

proper nutrition; an adequate supply of safe water and basic sanitation; maternal and child health care, including family planning; immunization against the major infectious diseases; prevention and control of locally endemic diseases; appropriate treatment of common diseases and injuries; and provision of essential drugs;

4. involves, in addition to the health sector, all related sectors and aspects of national and community development, in particular agriculture, animal husbandry, food, industry, education, housing, public works, communications and other sectors; and demands the coordinated efforts of all those sectors;

5. requires and promotes maximum community and individual self-reliance and participation in the planning, organization, operation and control of primary health care, making fullest use of local, national and other available resources; and to this end develops through appropriate education the ability of communities to participate;

6. should be sustained by integrated, functional and mutually-supportive referral systems, leading to the progressive improvement of comprehensive health care for all, and giving priority to those most in need;

7. relies, at local and referral levels, on health workers, including physicians, nurses, midwives, auxiliaries and community workers as applicable, as well as traditional practitioners as needed, suitably trained socially and technically to work as a health team and to respond to the expressed health needs of the community.

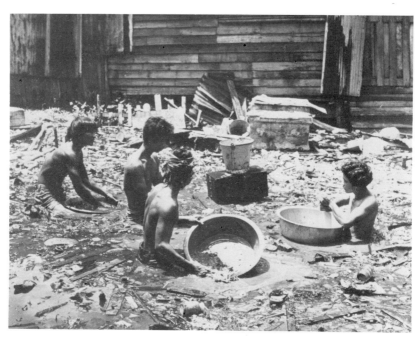

WHO Photo Competition: Ghulam Rasul Zafar

Environmental conditions have a major impact on health.

Since the Alma-Ata Conference, primary health care, in the words of another WHO document,[1] "has become the main thrust and focus for the promotion of world health . . . the dawn of a new vision about how to achieve better health for the people of the world."

Visions and ideals, of course, can, as the authors point out, be interpreted differently by different people and different countries, and in the ten years that have passed since the meeting in Alma-Ata, the meaning of the term "primary health care" has been considerably clarified.

The WHO Expert Committee Report, *Hospitals and health for all* (7), has this to say on the point:

Primary health care does not simply mean community health services or primary medical care in a conventional sense. It can be looked at in several different ways:

- as a range of programmes adapted to the patterns of health and disease of people living in a particular setting;
- as a level of care (the exact definition depending upon the country concerned) backed up by a well-organized referral system;
- as a strategy for reorienting the health system in order to provide the whole population with effective essential care, and to promote individual and community involvement and intersectoral collaboration; and
- as a philosophy, based on the principles of social equity, self-reliance, and community development.

Whichever way primary health care is looked at, hospital involvement is essential. If primary health care is regarded as a range of programmes, it requires the back-up of hospitals in promotive and preventive activities, as well as curative and rehabilitative services. If it is regarded as a level of care, primary health care will not work unless there is effective hospital support to deal with referred patients, and to refer patients who do not require hospital attention back to one of the other primary health care services. If it is regarded as a strategy it will not work without an adequate investment of skills and finance which, at present, are mainly in the hospital sector. Moreover, the philosophy of primary health care is just as relevant to what goes on within hospitals, as to what happens outside them.

This then is the sort of care that the Global Strategy for Health for All (adopted by the 34th World Health Assembly in 1981) is designed to turn from theory into reality in the near future.

Whether such an achievement is possible remains to be seen. As the *Hospitals and health for all* report (7) says:

---

[1] SMITH, D. L. ET AL. *Primary health care: A look at its meaning.* Unpublished WHO document, VBC/ECV/82.4.

To achieve the goal of health for all it is necessary to reorient the whole health system to meet new challenges through an integrated approach to the preventive, promotive, curative, and rehabilitative aspects of health care. This approach envisages the full involvement of hospitals in the planning and delivery of primary health care. It also implies a sharing between hospitals and other local health services of the responsibility for individual care at home, in the community, and at the first referral level.

Knowing how slowly health care systems, especially on a national basis, respond to change, it is indeed a mountainous task to accomplish a transformation of the type and the scale envisaged by the health for all concept. It would be foolish to overlook or underestimate the size and complexity of the job to be done. It would be equally foolish to forget that what moves mountains is faith.

Chapter 3. Origins

In Chapters 1 and 2, we made some suggestions as to the reasons for the reformation that is beginning to take place in the health services of the world: what we call the health care revolution. In this chapter we shall look briefly, but in a little more detail, at aspects of the changing times and of the changing circumstances of and attitudes to health care that may account for this remarkable occurrence.

Changing times

Major socioeconomic changes in the world reflect the spirit of the times during which they take place, and the features that seem particularly to have affected health care over recent years are, not unexpectedly, the development of space-age technology, the rise of what might be called "internationalism", and the march of medicine.

The technology of an age that has put men on the moon and satellites into space has made many marks on modern society, but none more obvious than the developments that have taken place in transportation and communications. Journeys that only forty years ago took weeks can now be completed in hours. Events taking place in one country today can be seen and heard in the homes of the inhabitants of others on the opposite side of the world while they are actually happening.

We are living in what is—to use a popular phrase—a shrinking world, and one in which it is now virtually impossible for any nation to remain isolated from the changes taking place around it.

The world is becoming more genuinely "international" than ever before, a trend much influenced and hastened by the existence of the United Nations Organization. The UN was established in October 1945, as a direct consequence of two world wars having taken place in less than a quarter of a century. A "parliament for the world", it was designed to try to keep the peace through its Security Council and to improve living standards for all people of the world by means of campaigns against poverty and disease mounted via its Economic and Social Council.

One of the major specialized agencies of the UN is, of course, the World Health Organization, prime mover in the campaign for Health for All by the Year 2000, and originator of the Global Strategy by means of which the aim will, it is hoped, be achieved.

This campaign is a direct outcome of the march of modern medicine, a phenomenon that started at the turn of the century and which has grown apace over the past fifty years. An important characteristic of WHO's international concept, like many national activities that have been undertaken in the health care field in recent years, is neither to hasten nor to slow the march of scientific medicine but to deflect it on to a course that will be of maximum benefit to the health of the people of the world and in line with the changing circumstances of the international health care scene.

Changing circumstances

As Roberts suggested in 1952 (8), no nation on earth could afford any longer to finance all the aspirations of its medical practitioners or satisfy the great expectations that these create in the minds of the people.

"Medicine" he wrote "is advancing more rapidly than the capacity of statesmen and administrators to deal with it . . . The increasing cost of ill health, which had set in long before the inception [in 1948] of the [British] National Health Service, is due primarily and paradoxically to the advancement of medicine, which is spurred to perpetual acceleration by the perpetual acceleration of scientific discovery. To this process there can be no end, except that which is imposed by limitations in the available resources."

26

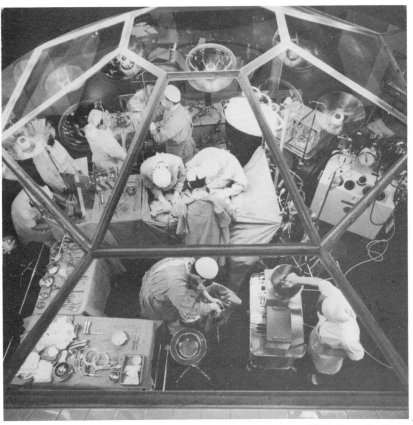

WHO Photo: P. Almasy

Expensive interventions contribute to the ever-increasing cost of health care.

Few, if any, students of health care today would disagree with that view. Every industrialized country has by now experienced the twin misfortunes of rapidly rising health care costs and a sluggish or even falling economic productivity.

Government intervention in the arrangements for the provision of health care to the people has increased. Even in that bastion of private enterprise, the United States of America, governmental payments for medical care provided to elderly and indigent sick people have become more restricted and circumscribed by the application of a prospective payment system, based on the classification of patients according to diagnosis and use of resources (diagnosis-related groups).

Similarly, other changes in legislation, demographic and social characteristics and morbidity patterns continue to affect health care systems. Social legislation regarding matters such as maternity leave, the liberty of the individual, sexual equality, confidentiality of information, and the length of the working week all affect costs and ways of working both in the health care field and outside it. Changing patterns of morbidity and demography— reduced fertility, increased life expectancy, unemployment, etc.—also have a significant impact on health care systems.

Hospital practice in all countries has been much affected in recent years by the changing sociodemographic and financial circumstances. In the more affluent days of twenty or thirty years ago, hospitals accepted patients who might more appropriately have been treated elsewhere. They were not especially cost-conscious institutions in an era when charges were retrospectively recoverable from governments, insurance companies and other sources.

Today, when such payments are often prospective, standardized, and limited, care and treatment must be seen to be appropriate to the level of the health care system involved (i.e., the hospital) as the emphasis on proven value for money and formal quality assurance grows.

In the USA, for example, hospitals are confronted by a variety of developments—the introduction of diagnosis-related groups; day surgery and therapy; and a growing demand for home care.

As one writer has commented:[1]

> [Home care] is part of an overall revolution in health services. It is not the only alternative to the hospital and, in fact, would fail if it tried to be. But as a sensitive part of a complex of inter-related services, e.g. primary care, acute care and chronic care, it has significant potential.

Under existing conditions, therefore, the noble ideal of a free and comprehensive health service, such as was envisaged for the United Kingdom in 1948, is one that no country

---

[1] McNERNEY, W. J., *The rationale for siting advanced health technologies at home.* Unpublished WHO document, SHS/EC/85/RPII.C.1.

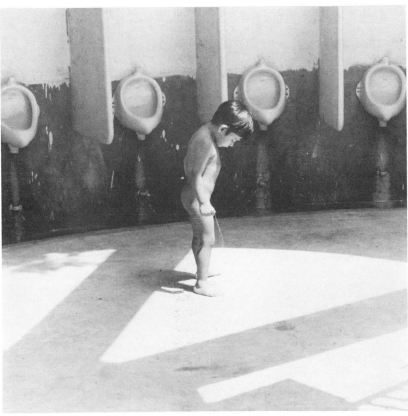

WHO Photo Competition: Dilip Chatterjee

Provisions must be appropriate to needs.

has yet been able to attain. The challenge, therefore, that all nations now face if they have any pretension to the provision of an equitable health care system to the whole population, is, in the words of Dr Roberts, "*not* a dedication to build the finest service in the world but to something infinitely higher; to the exercise of restraint and unselfishness whereby every person-identifies the interests of his fellows with his own" (*8*). It is a concept of a national health service very much in line with the WHO health for all philosophy.

Changing attitudes

In 1973 Professor Henry Miller, then Vice Chancellor of the University of Newcastle-upon-Tyne, England, had this to say about medicine and developing countries (9):

Contemporary medical research is particularly concerned with the investigation of the subtle factors that underlie such intractable disease as multiple sclerosis, cancer of the breast, and hypertension. But looked at in a global context these are insignificant by comparison with the malnutrition, the persistence of infections and infestations that we have controlled in the affluent societies but which, in Africa, Asia, and Latin America, mean that half of all deaths occur in children under 5. . . .

A further problem is of course that the export of modern therapeutics to the third world has been unsupported by two other developments that would enhance its benefits and diminish its dangers: the simultaneous export of measures to control the population explosion, and of the knowledge and machinery to furnish an agricultural and industrial infrastructure without which it will never be able to sustain the heavy real cost of modern medicine. In the meantime, millions of people all over the world die every year from diseases that can and could be controlled on the basis of existing knowledge and of techniques that are well within our grasp . . . The dangers implicit in the division between the rich and poor countries of the world pose a greater threat to the future of human civilization than the possibility of destruction by nuclear weapons, and it is important that the medical aspects of the situation should be fully realized. The important decisions to be taken are on the scale of world politics, but the contribution of medicine is essential: it could be central and immensely important.

These of course are the views of a medical academic, but they are in step with those of the World Health Assemblies of the early 1970s which stressed the need for change in the way health services were then (and in varying ways still are) provided, as a matter of vital international importance.

Included in a report on the need to develop basic health services throughout the world, which was made to the Executive Board of the World Health Organization in 1973, was an appreciation of the then existing position (3). It advanced the following opinions.

The Board is of the opinion that in many countries the health services are not keeping pace with the changing populations either in quantity or in quality. It is likely that they are getting worse. Even if this is looked at optimistically and it is said that the health services are improving, the Board considers that a major crisis is on the point of developing and that it must ' be faced at once, as it could result in a reaction that could be both destructive and costly. There appears to be widespread dissatisfaction of populations about their health services for varying reasons. Such dissatisfaction occurs in the developed as well as in the third world. The causes can be summarized as a failure to meet the expectations of the populations; an inability of the health services to deliver a level of national coverage adequate to meet the stated demands and the changing needs of different societies; a wide gap (which is not closing) in health status between countries, and between different groups within countries; rapidly rising costs without a visible and meaningful improvement in service; and a feeling of helplessness on the part of the consumer, who feels (rightly or wrongly) that the health services and the personnel within them are progressing along an uncontrollable path of their own which may be satisfying to the health professions but which is not what is most wanted by the consumer. . .

Many other factors responsible for the present position could be listed. It is not considered that any one predominates or that it can explain most of what is happening. Most are correctable and all deserve detailed attention. Rather it is appropriate to state that they are possibly symptoms of a wide and deep-seated error in the way health services are provided.

Of course, this view was not a new one. The Health Organization of the League of Nations was saying much the same thing fifty years ago.

An Intergovernmental Conference of Far Eastern Countries on Rural Hygiene, which met in Java in 1937 (*10*), concluded that the key to a better quality of life for the world's poor and disadvantaged rural people was the provision of better, decentralized health services which the local communities would accept because they would be freely involved in deciding the form of their organization and content.

"The opening of public health work in rural areas," the Conference suggested, "can often be used as the entering wedge for the development of a broader programme embracing education, economics, sociology, engineering and agriculture . . . [such work must be based on] the cooperation of the people at the periphery."

The conclusions of this largely forgotten Conference are not just of historical interest, they are apposite to the subject of this chapter, for they are much akin to the proposals put by the Director-General of WHO, Dr Halfdan Mahler, to the 28th World Health Assembly in 1975—the occasion when the Assembly adopted the concept of primary health care (PHC) and so gave official recognition and approval at the highest international level of health care deliberation, to the need for, and the form of, a worldwide health care revolution. As Dr Mahler wrote later (*11*):

In my paper to the Assembly[1] PHC was characterized by the following seven principles:

(a) Primary health care should be shaped around the life patterns of the population it should serve and should meet the needs of the community.

(b) Primary health care should be an integral part of the national health system, and other echelons of services should be designed in support of the needs of the peripheral level, especially as this pertains to technical supply, supervisory and referral support.

(c) Primary health care activities should be fully integrated with the activities of the other sectors involved in community development (agriculture, education, public works, housing, communications).

(d) The local population should be actively involved in the formulation and implementation of health care activities so that health care can be brought into line with local needs and priorities. Decisions upon what are the community needs requiring solution should be based upon a continuing dialogue between the people and the services.

(e) The health care offered should place maximum reliance on the available community resources, especially those which have hitherto remained untapped, and should remain within the stringent cost limitations that are present in each country.

(f) Primary health care should use an integrated approach of preventive, promotive, curative and rehabilitative services for the individual, family and community. The balance between these services should vary according to community needs and may well change over time.

(g) The majority of health interventions should be undertaken at the most peripheral practicable level of the health services by workers most suitably trained for performing these activities.

I also emphasized that no single model of PHC exists which has general applicability. Each of the seven principles listed can be translated into action in countless ways; the important thing is that these ways should evolve from and reflect the *unique* aspects of national values, conditions, and lifestyles.

The similarity between these principles and the conclusions reached in 1937 cannot be denied.

But why did WHO, in 1975, need to reaffirm proposals put forward forty years earlier? Why had these proposals not already been implemented, especially since they were based on international agreement? Why, in Dr Mahler's words, had "the commitment to an intersectoral approach to health, founded upon an active involvement of the people" not been adhered to?

There are, of course, a variety of reasons, some of which have been suggested in the previous chapter.

---

[1] WHO document A28/9.

Regrettable though the delay in implementation has been, more important today is the decision of the 1975 World Health Assembly to go ahead with the promotion of primary health care.

As Dr Mahler put it:

More important is the necessity to reconsider the strategy that we have chosen. Rather than decry the sad state we are in, I believe we must work toward health as a social goal, and we must assess developments in the light of their ability to contribute to this goal. In characterizing primary health care the way we have, we are putting it forward as an alternative to the dominating trends of the past few decades. It is an alternative that has more than once been recognized as the best road to take, but somehow the choice has always been made for other ways. Now I believe it is no longer an alternative: it is an imperative.

The necessity to proceed with implementing primary health care is part of a wider necessity to seek social justice. The forces that confined progress in the health sector to a few persons have also ignored the many needs that require satisfaction if human well-being is to be achieved. The importance that primary health care gives to community involvement is part of a greater need for individuals, families, and communities to be the prime movers in all aspects of their own development, not just health. The failure to achieve equitable development has rested largely on the isolation of people from decision-making processes and on the erection of independent sectoral bureaucracies which have little contact with reality. Even the call for "community development" some 30 to 40 years ago became the work of the bureaucracy alone, rather than that of the people. Other sectors have come to similar conclusions and are pressing for similar programs in their respective areas of influence.

When Dr Mahler wrote these words, some interesting examples of what could be achieved by dedicated people working largely in poor rural areas of developing countries had already been described in *Health by the people* (*12*), edited by Kenneth W. Newell, then Director of the Division of Strengthening of Health Services at WHO Headquarters in Geneva.

The book included reports of non-hospital and largely non-medical projects that had significantly improved the health care of rural people in nine countries—China, Cuba, Guatemala, India, Indonesia, the Islamic Republic of Iran, Niger, the United Republic of Tanzania, and Venezuela. As Dr Newell wrote:

My reaction on reading these accounts was one of excitement. Excitement that such victories in the health field have been won in many geographical regions, in countries with widely different political systems, and in some of

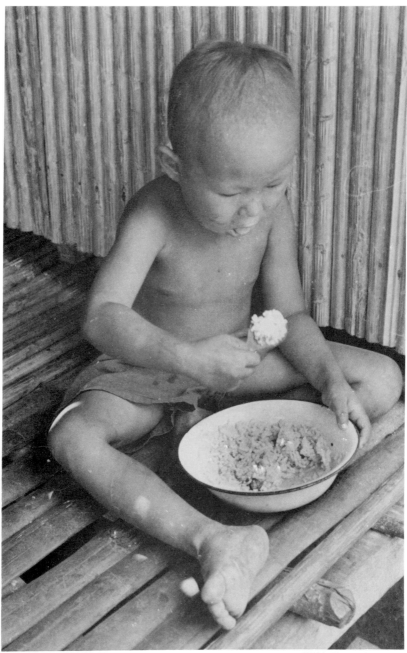

WHO Photo: Gramiccia

Adequate nutrition is a prerequisite for health.

34

the poorest rural populations of the world. By the use of well-accepted—almost conventional—simple health techniques and the provision of food, education, and assistance in improving productivity, the health of communities has improved dramatically and visibly and in a way that makes one optimistic about the potential for continuing change.

This view is strongly reinforced by Sanders & Carver in their book, *The struggle for health* (4), where they point out that the success stories of better health in underdeveloped countries have had more to do with changed economic and political systems and improved nutrition, water provision, and sanitation than with technological modern medicine.

The two most important measures to promote health in the countries that are now developed were improved nutrition and better environmental hygiene. Exactly the same measures are needed to promote health in underdeveloped countries today. But the task of ending underdevelopment is not just a repetition of the development that took place in Britain and the other advanced capitalist countries. We have seen how the accumulation of capital for industrial development in those countries came from exploiting the colonial world. The underdeveloped countries today have no colonies to exploit—they have no easy source of capital and only small markets for their goods. Since the advent of imperialism, the economies of underdeveloped countries have become increasingly controlled by huge foreign-owned enterprises in alliance with a local ruling class.

The possibility of significant independent capitalist development as happened in nineteenth-century Europe no longer exists. There are, however, a few impressive examples of countries where underdevelopment is being successfully tackled and great improvements in their people's health achieved. The best known of these are Cuba and China where victorious popular struggles resulted in a change of economic and political systems. Long-stifled human potential was mobilized, foreign-controlled resources reappropriated and the ensuing wealth more fairly distributed, with particular emphasis on health and other social services.

35

Chapter 4. The hospital function at the first referral level

This chapter and the next are concerned with two essential elements of the ideology of the health care revolution: the integration of hospital and primary health care services and the establishment of a system of care based in health districts.

What we are concerned to emphasize here is the elementary but fundamental fact that hospital and primary health care services are two inter-related and equally necessary parts of a truly comprehensive system of health care provision. Neither can operate properly without the other, and to consider them as separate and opposing entities rather than as a single one is, in the words of a WHO Expert Committee (7), a false antithesis, common and of long standing, and with "enough semblance of the truth to be thoroughly dangerous".

For as the Committee went on to say, whichever way primary health care is looked at—as a range of programmes, a level of care, a strategy for reorienting the health system, or a philosophy of provision—hospital involvement is essential.

And that involvement must include *all* hospitals, whether local, regional or national; whether providing primary, secondary or tertiary care; and whether owned and operated by government, charity, or for-profit organizations.

Each must play its part in an integrated and comprehensive service for the simple reason that if it does not then the total service will be out of balance and will not serve the people to the best advantage. All hospitals are therefore affected by the health care revolution, although in this chapter we are specifically concerned with those that function as first referral level hospitals, whether or not they also offer secondary and/or tertiary level care.

But what are the role and functions of the hospital at the first referral level?

The WHO Expert Committee considered this question in some detail and came to the conclusion that such hospitals had specific responsibilities in support of primary health care in four main areas: direct patient care, health programme coordination, education and training, and management and administrative support.

Direct patient care

The direct care and treatment of individual patients is, in theory, a relatively straightforward matter. The patient is referred to the hospital by the appropriate primary health worker when the primary health care facilities are inadequate for the patient. The hospital at the first referral level then assesses the patient's condition in the light of the information provided by the primary health care service, and either treats him directly or passes him on for further examination and/or treatment at the secondary or tertiary level. The patient is subsequently discharged back to the primary care level with details of care given and further care required.

The mechanics of the system are the same everywhere. Their practical application to individual patients will differ widely in different locations depending on the completeness and quality of the total health service available, the availability of other public services, the standards of living and education of the people concerned, and a variety of other geographical, social, and political factors.

Even if all the elements of an integrated health service are technically in place, the system can still be easily upset by problems of self-referral by patients who have little faith in anything but hospital care; by inappropriate referral by inexperienced or overworked primary health care workers; by inappropriate or misguided hospital treatment; or by the provision of inadequate referral or discharge information.

For this reason, an essential part of the health care revolution is the coordination of hospital and primary health care activities.

Health programme coordination

The report, *Hospitals and health for all* (7), includes a conceptual model of a comprehensive health system based on the principles of primary health care as shown in Fig. 1.

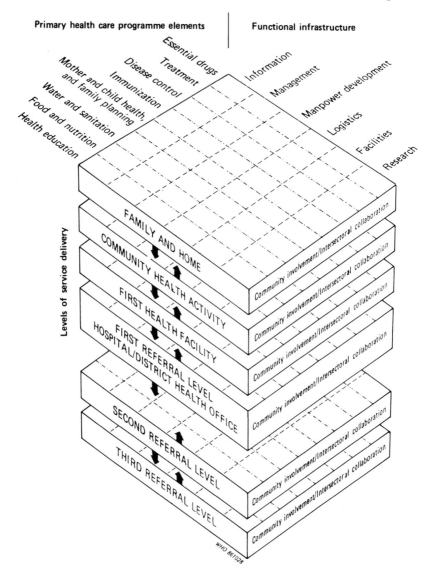

Fig. 1. A conceptual model of a comprehensive health system based on the principles of primary health care

The model is conceptually simple but, because it is represented in three dimensions, is visually somewhat complex.

It is presented as a box to indicate resource and other limitations inherent in all defined populations, irrespective of the actual level of resources. The box appears to contain many separate little blocks, all vitally interconnected, with the levels of service delivery, the elements of the primary health care programmes, and the infrastructure determinants set out on the three dimensions. As can be seen from the drawing, these three dimensions must be perceived as operating on the basis of community involvement, intersectoral collaboration and concern for appropriate technology.

The model sets out both the components of primary care and the interactions of these components with hospitals— especially with hospitals providing a first referral level service, i.e., those that have the necessary staff, resources and organization to undertake more complicated medical activities and invasive treatments than are available at the first health facility level.

It also illustrates the fundamental fact that to improve health, the whole of the box—not just one section of it— must grow and expand, and that when considering the development of any section, the possible effects (whether good or bad) of such a development on other sections, must be taken into account.

Finally, the model makes it quite clear that if hospitals are genuinely to help improve people's health, they cannot work in isolation but must cooperate and be concerned with all the other providers of health care in the community, whether in government or nongovernmental organizations, and whether health workers or civic groups with an interest in health. Figure 2 shows how the model fits into a health infrastructure based on primary health care.

The Expert Committee, when commenting on the model, had this to say on the need for, and on ways of achieving, health programme coordination:

Apart from the treatment of individual patients, hospitals should be involved in the planning, coordination, and evaluation of the implementation of the main elements of primary health care (see the face of the model . . . . labelled primary health care programme elements). They can play a role in at least four types of programme concerned with these main elements:

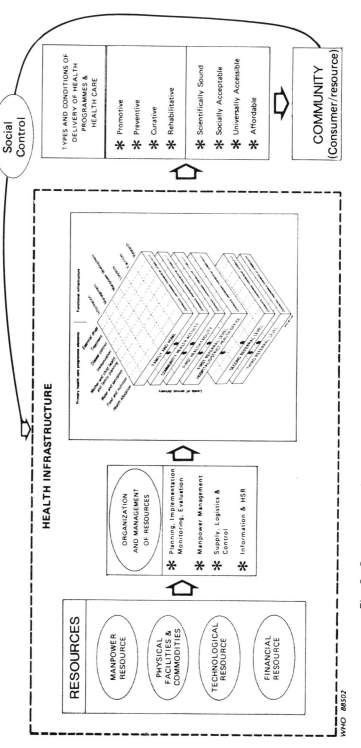

Fig. 2. Components of a comprehensive health system based on primary health care

WHO 88502

- programmes confined to hospital patients and their families, such as health education in the hospital;
- single-function or special-focus primary health care programmes such as nutrition, maternal and child care, immunization, rabies prevention, or mental health;
- comprehensive primary health care programmes, for example, when hospitals are given responsibility for total health care within a specified geographical area; and
- community development programmes, including comprehensive actions to promote health.

While, ideally, disease-specific programmes should not be conceived or implemented in isolation, there is no doubt that they can be extremely effective. Malnutrition, water contamination, or infectious diseases of childhood are examples of specific health problems that can be tackled by implementing targeted programmes, i.e., by deciding what to do, mobilizing the resources to do it, and gauging the effect. It is easy enough to see that the hospital at the first referral level often has a contribution to make to such programmes. In nutrition, for example, this would include carrying out diagnostic tests (such as serum protein tests and tests to determine the extent of anaemia), counselling, and treating referred cases. The hospital's contribution could also embrace a much wider range of nutrition-related activities, such as educational and logistic support for health professionals and community health workers, and the analysis of survey data. Quite obviously, the hospital's contribution will be of limited, even negligible, value if all it does is treat referred patients without reference to the root causes of malnutrition in the community and to the environment to which its patients return after they are discharged. Thus, the hospital must become involved at the most fundamental level of health promotion and disease prevention.

This example is only one among many: effective programmes for obstetric, neonatal, and paediatric care all provide incontrovertible evidence of the essential interdependence between community-based and hospital-based activities. For every obstetric or neonatal emergency requiring sophisticated intervention, many more will respond to first-line measures in the home or health centre. Outreach from the hospital is essential if these problems are to be dealt with effectively. Moreover, it is important that those at risk are recognized and that, when hospital referral is warranted, it takes place in time, with appropriate care meanwhile. It is equally important that the hospital-based obstetrics team knows the facts and the circumstances of birth and birth-related mortality and morbidity in the population it serves. Unfortunately, district hospitals often lack this information. Because baseline information is seldom available, district hospitals are unable to evaluate progress in reducing morbidity and mortality. Generally speaking, district hospital staff are preoccupied with their daily caseload of patients and work in isolation from events in the community outside.

Further examples of the need to relate what the hospital does to what goes on outside its walls could be provided in relation to diarrhoeal diseases, mental illness, mental and physical handicap, the care of the elderly, etc. In all these fields, the only approach to health care that makes sense is a community-based service, with hospital promotive, preventive, and curative activities as an integral component. Moreover, from work in such fields as these come particular insights into the importance of emotional, psychological, and cultural sensitivity when dealing with "other people's" problems, which should influence all health programmes.

Education and training

Manifestly hospitals can be—and often are—excellent centres for the provision of health education and training of both staff and public. Examples of this were given in Chapter 1, which also noted that such activities need to encompass other institutions and organizations—from farms to employment agencies—that are not usually seen as part of the health system.

Hospitals must obviously ensure that their own staff are properly educated and trained to understand and play their continuing part in primary health care, just as they must participate in the basic and further training of all health workers in their district.

There is also no reason why, within the context of the local health district (see Chapter 5), the hospital should not provide the base for more advanced professional education and for the development of senior staff, through management and leadership training, to administer the district service on the basis of the primary health care philosophy.

Management and administrative support

If limited health care resources are to be used effectively to serve the interests of sick people, good management of those resources is vital.

In the conceptual model of a comprehensive health system, reproduced on page 38, management's direct and oblique participation in the operation of the system is shown in what is called the "functional infrastructure" dimension.

The report of the WHO Expert Committee (7) comments upon the managerial and administrative input to the health system as follows:

Managerial and logistic interactions of various kinds form an important part of the relationship between the hospital at the first referral level and other local health services . . . . The degree of hospital involvement in management depends on whether (a) the hospital is organizationally separate from the rest of the district health system, (b) there is a separate district health office that manages the district health system as a whole, or (c) the headquarters of the health service is based within the hospital. If the headquarters is based in the hospital, then it must not be hospital-dominated, since supporting and directing the whole complex web of primary health care activities calls for insight, sensitivity, and skills that have little to do with the traditional roles of hospitals. Included within the range of management functions are resource allocation and control; intersectoral action for health; manpower development and deployment; purchasing and distribution of supplies; and planning, monitoring, and evaluation of the health status and health services based on an effective information system and on research.

But having considered the first referral level hospital function in theory, how might the theory appear in practice? One informed critic has made the following suggestions (13):

In the world's more than 100 developing countries today, first level referral support by small community hospitals is essential to the success of primary health care. Consequently, there must be a national commitment to build an infrastructure of supportive curative services. One approach would be to upgrade some of the primary health care centres, by adding modern facilities, so as to provide basic supportive services in the major branches of medicine. Such a centre should then be capable of diagnosing and treating a case of cerebral malaria with proper diagnostic verification; diagnosing and treating a case of small bowel obstruction in a child, where the major problem is roundworm blocking the gut; evacuating a uterus with retained placenta in a mother who might otherwise bleed to death; treating a patient with severe third degree burns, providing adequate fluid and electrolyte replacement to prevent over-hydration or under-hydration, and covering the areas with skin graft when appropriate; saving the life of a young child with diphtheria by doing a tracheotomy; giving advice to a mother on oral rehydration if a child is brought in with early signs of dehydration, or if necessary admitting the child for proper nursing care and oral rehydration, if so desired; or excising all dead tissue in a compound comminuted fracture of the tibia and providing adequate protection to the limb to save it, maintain its length and let the fracture heal.

These are just examples among an extensive list of medical, surgical, gynaecological and paediatric conditions which are daily occurrences, and where a small hospital must be capable of diagnosing early, treating adequately and producing good enough results to win the institution a sound reputation among the local public. This is particularly true when communities are isolated and scattered; in such circumstances, having to travel to a city hospital would not only involve costly long-distance transport but also late arrivals and unnecessary complications, possibly resulting in loss of life or limb.

Manifestly, however, the practice is not always successful, for as the same writer goes on to say:

In many countries of the developing world, such small hospitals do exist at the periphery and they have been doing excellent work. Quite frequently they have been aided by foreign charities or religious missions. Sometimes they grew out of local enthusiasm and the loving labour of a dedicated physician.

At the same time, many of the hospitals that have developed out of so-called upgraded primary health centres lack both manpower and material. Doctors posted to such institutions too often regard their work as drudgery, and thus fail to build up the local community's confidence in their skill. They may be under-paid, their children have little or no educational facilities, and they yearn to be posted back to the big cities in a public health service system. Drugs are inadequately supplied or even non-existent, and working conditions are uncomfortable.

Chapter 5. The district health system

What exactly constitutes a district health system and why should it be considered as essential to the sort of health care revolution we are considering? After all, a number of countries already organize their health services on a district basis without necessarily demonstrating any special enthusiasm or support in practice for the primary health care approach.

One such country is the United Kingdom. It has had a National Health Service organized on a district and regional basis for more than a decade. In addition, the health authorities that now administer the service were officially asked some years ago by the Department of Health and Social Security in London to encourage the development of health promotion, community-based care, and other similar primary health care policies (*14*). However, the progress made so far has been small and slow.

Nevertheless, there are very good reasons why health care should be greatly improved by being organized and provided on a district health system basis, as expounded in the **WHO** Expert Committee report on *Hospitals and health for all* (*7*).

First of all, however, what do we mean by a district health system?

A district health system based on primary health care comprises first and foremost a well-defined population, living within a clearly delineated administrative and geographical area, whether urban or rural. It includes all the relevant health care agencies in the area, whether governmental or independent, professional or traditional, which cooperate to create a district system and work together within it. A district health system therefore consists of a large variety of interrelated elements that contribute to health in homes, schools, work places, and communities, and is multisectoral in orientation. It includes self-care and all health care workers and facilities, whether governmental or non-governmental, up to and including the hospital at the first referral level, and the appropriate support services, such as laboratory, diagnostic, and logistic support. It needs to be managed as a single entity, normally under a single full-time manager who has public health as well as curative responsibilities, in order to draw together all these elements and institutions into a fully comprehensive range of promotive, preventive, curative, and rehabilitative health activities, and to monitor progress.

Substantial managerial authority should be delegated to the district health system by government and others in order that decisions can, as far as possible, be taken within the district, with the active involvement of those who live there. The aim of a district health system is to combine the coordinated efforts of all the relevant elements and institutions in pursuit of health for all.

Key features of the district health system are that:

- it is people-centred, emphasizing all the health-related elements of their behaviour and their environment, and their right to shape their own health care with professional help;
- it is based, whenever possible, on a discrete geographical area, within clearly delineated boundaries, and includes the whole population within that area and all health care workers and facilities up to and including the hospital at the first referral level;
- it need not be exclusively a government system, and may be composed of many elements, including, for example, non-governmental institutions and traditional healers;
- it has substantial managerial autonomy in order to be able to settle priorities and problems, as far as possible, on a decentralized basis; and
- it incorporates the primary health care approach into all its activities.

As for the reason why the district health system is an essential element in the ideology of the health care revolution—firstly there is the question of implementing the declaration of Alma-Ata.

The Expert Committee emphasized that all the services that contribute to primary health care should be oriented towards serving a defined population. Unless this is the case, it is hard to see how the precepts of Alma-Ata can be put into practice, particularly the pursuit of universal health coverage, the assessment of health needs and the impact of services, and community participation in the management of health care institutions.

Secondly, there is the need to have a concept of overall health care that is not only comprehensible but capable of being introduced in practice. The provision of a complete service to a given number of people in a defined geographical area is a sensible and demonstrable way of achieving this.

The district provides a framework within which to think coherently about the hospital in relation to the people whom it serves, and in relation to all the other relevant agencies, including those not usually considered as part of the health sector.

Thirdly, an international reform of health care provision, of the sort we have in mind, is just not possible unless hospitals can be encouraged to review and revise their activities in the light of the total health needs of the people.

Without studying a defined population, the hospital at the first referral level cannot critically examine its own performance in the context of other health services. For example, an examination of the role of hospitals in Pelotas, Rio Grande do Sul, Brazil, in 1982, showed that antenatal care was inversely correlated with risk, and that caesarean sections were positively correlated with family income rather than with risk. Thus, neither the poor nor the rich received optimal care: the first group received too little, and the latter too much. Inadequate and inappropriate treatment of this kind may well go unrecognized unless the work of hospitals is studied in the broad context of community needs and other health care provision.

To know what a district health system is and why it is important for the future development of health care services worldwide is, however, only the first small step towards creating such a system. The obstacles that lie between the conception and its implementation are formidable and should not be underestimated.

To start with, getting hospital staff to change their ways of working is likely to be no easy matter.

It can be extraordinarily difficult to direct the activities of the hospital to meet the specific needs of the population it serves. This is especially so where hospital resources are small and where the population is widely dispersed. For example, the Patan Hospital, Nepal (which serves a population of 210 000) finds it exceedingly difficult to provide effective support to health posts that are up to two days' journey from the hospital, and equally difficult to avoid becoming wholly absorbed in providing services for those who happen to live close by, even though there is no real need in most cases for hospital treatment. This problem is also recognized in Kasongo, Zaire, where unnecessary hospital treatment of this type is seen as an "operational loophole" to be worked out of the system if the hospital is to concentrate on its referral functions.

In some countries it is accepted practice to refer patients to the particular hospital that serves their neighbourhood, but in many others the patient and the referring practitioner can choose to use another hospital if it is preferred. The right to refer across boundaries is often seen as an important protection against bureaucracy, and it would be sad to see such freedom eliminated. Nevertheless, it is reasonable to encourage, rather than discourage, rational patterns of referral; for example, by giving patients referred from remote health posts preference at the hospital over self-referred patients so that they are seen more quickly and by a specialist, if necessary. Charges also are important since many patients are reluctant to incur additional expense. In Kasongo, Zaire, referral and hospitalization charges are included in the initial fee paid by the patients at the health centre.

Then there is the question of integration and the achievement of full cooperation between hospitals and primary health care and other services, without which a comprehensive district health system cannot be established.

A survey carried out in 14 countries in tropical Africa by the Royal Tropical Institute, Amsterdam, showed that the majority (approximately 75%) of the hospitals that responded had formal referral arrangements with health centres, dispensaries, or village health workers. In many respects, however, the contacts fell short of a close partnership and suggested far too narrow an understanding of primary health care. For example, only about 50% collected health data at the village level, and only 60% involved local communities in any way in health decisions.

Effective cooperation is of course harder to achieve in situations where hospitals and other institutions and health care workers that comprise a district health system, work within separate organizations, and are separately funded and controlled.

The Expert Committee considered that the variations in economic, social, and political settings were too great for it to be able to describe an ideal district health system, although models exist in, for example, China, India, the United Kingdom, and the USSR. The Committee was firmly of the opinion that every hospital at the first referral level should be linked to a defined population, and have a special commitment to the health of the community that it serves and to other local health services and health workers in its area. Whenever possible, the population it serves should be geographically defined. In urban areas with many hospitals, there are special problems that may be best resolved by some form of consortium, rather than by seeking to create artificial boundaries. Even if a hospital does not have a major role in clinical referral at the first level, it should have a role in promoting primary health care for its patients and their families. Even hospitals at the second and third referral level may, by agreement, become involved in primary health care (particularly for the purposes of treating patients, teaching, and research), but they would have to learn how to discharge this role well, and to hold it in balance with their other activities. Where primary health care is weak, hospitals may have a role in reaching out to strengthen or even to help create it.

Finally, the district health system concept, like the philosophy of health for all through the promotion of primary health care itself, is based on the assumption that the people who comprise the health district will be intimately involved in determining the type and level of health services provided, and the ways they are provided.

"The people", said the Declaration of Alma-Ata, "have the right and duty to participate individually and collectively in the planning and implementation of their health care."

"Health", the report of the WHO Expert Committee propounded, "can never be adequately protected by health services without the active understanding and involvement of the individuals and communities whose health is at stake. Action to promote health therefore depends on a partnership based on mutual understanding and trust, between those working in the health sector and the community."

However, it is notoriously difficult to bring about satisfactory and effective community involvement in health care planning and provision. As an example from an industrialized country, the Community Health Councils (one for each Health District) specially set up in the United Kingdom to achieve such cooperation, have had limited success for a variety of reasons, of which one is undoubtedly public apathy.

As the Expert Committee commented:

> The need for community involvement applies to hospitals as much as to any other part of the health system. However, community involvement is not easy to achieve as extensive experience has indicated.[1] . . . Among the reasons given for this are that people have not always been encouraged to think and choose for themselves, and have therefore become used to 'solutions' being imposed upon them by experts. In addition, not enough effort and imagination have been devoted to structuring the health service in such a way that people can participate in more than just token ways. Among the key issues of community involvement are: the kind of participation that should be sought to achieve specific goals; who should participate; and the type and method of participation.[1] Some radical changes in thinking are required in the community, as well as among health professionals, if individually and collectively people are to take responsibility for their own health. The role of the experts should be to provide information and support, so that individuals and communities can decide what *they* want.

Notwithstanding these strictures, there are many welcome signs in many countries that inter-relationships and interconnections between hospitals and the communities they exist to serve, are beginning to broaden and strengthen. We are aware, for example, of attempts to create district health services under difficult conditions in Siddarjo, Indonesia; Suihua, China; Santa Cruz, Philippines; Upazila, Bangladesh; and Hurungwe, Zimbabwe. And in the United Kingdom, projects based on health for all principles are being undertaken in a number of health districts (*15, 16*).

The final extract from the WHO Expert Committee report has been chosen because, in addition to offering some

---

[1] *Community involvement in health systems for primary health care.* Unpublished WHO document, SHS/83.69.

further explanations for the lack of hospital–community links in most countries, and making sensible suggestions for remedying the situation, it also gives further examples (some of which we have already quoted) of how the problems have been successfully overcome. It is fitting that this chapter should end on an encouraging note.

On the whole, hospitals have lagged behind other sectors of the health service in terms of community involvement; there are all sorts of explanation, such as overemphasis on the disease model of hospital care and the lack of contact with a defined community. However, these attitudes must change if hospitals are to play their proper role in primary health care; comprehensive care that includes both prevention and treatment is essential. Moreover, with resources becoming increasingly scarce, hospitals have no right to decide for the communities that they serve which health issues should be given priority; technical decisions are one thing, but choices of priority are generally at least as much social and political as technical.

The need for real community involvement provides one good argument for the definition of the population to be served by each hospital at the first referral level, since this would at least make it clear which community should be involved.

Greater decentralization of government than now exists may be required for community involvement to be worthwhile. Initially, community leaders are often sceptical that central government will recognize their contribution to health care, and are quite right not to waste their time unless their involvement will pay off for their community. The interest of local communities goes beyond health services alone, and thus they should be able to insist upon intersectoral collaboration.

Hospitals are not remote like some institutions of government. Communities readily identify with them and they have substantial prestige and a position of leadership in most communities (as do the hospital-based medical and nursing staff). If hospitals and their professional staffs are serious about community involvement, that will itself influence the community's response.

This is also true of health education and health promotion. For many health problems (ranging from malnutrition to heart disease, and from alcoholism and violence to loss of independence in old age), hospital care is not an adequate or effective response. Hospitals have their part to play in health education and health promotion and their example will be important.

Paradoxically, while independent hospitals may in many cases seem less closely linked to other health services in the locality and to specific catchment populations than state hospitals, they may also be less constrained by central regulations. They may therefore be in a particularly good position to initiate community involvement.

Despite real difficulties, there are some encouraging examples of community involvement in hospitals, and of hospital involvement in community development and health promotion, in many parts of the world. In China, for example, there are direct links between health agencies at each level and community councils or committees that ensure intersectoral coordination, and although the mechanisms and traditions are different, the same is true in the USSR. In many other parts of the world, the examples are of single institutions rather than whole systems: for instance, in the neighbourhood ('patch-based') projects and the 'hospitals without walls' in Costa Rica, and in hospital-based projects in Hong Kong, New York, and Sierra Leone.

Chapter 6. Problems of implementation: organizational and functional integration of services

Reviewing the situation

In previous chapters we have propounded the view that throughout the world there is a growing awareness of a need for change in order that health services may match more closely the needs of the people. We have said that we see this "health care revolution" as epitomized in and inspired by the WHO Global Strategy for Health for All by the Year 2000.

We have given reasons why a development of this kind should have manifested itself at the present time, and have suggested that the reformed and truly democratic health care system envisaged will operate best on the basis of relatively small health districts, each providing a full range of primary health care services closely integrated with hospital services through a local institution performing the first referral level hospital function.

But we would be the first to admit that *wanting* a new system of health care provision and *creating* such a system throughout the world are two very different things.

Even when a hospital is built to support an already existing and growing community primary health care programme, as was the case with the Patan Hospital in Nepal (mentioned in Chapter 1), the practical problems of achieving the necessary integration of services are considerable. You will recall the hospital medical director's comment on this point.

This is a world of trial, experience, and modification, of successes and failures. Satisfactory approaches at a given time and in a given situation may not work at another time or in another place.

The health care revolution therefore is not likely to happen quickly. It will of necessity be a gradual development, owing as much to the evolution of ideas as to the revolution of practice. Progress is likely to consist of an accretion of innumerable small advances.

Nevertheless, it will happen, because throughout the world, in every country, health workers are already experimenting with their particular health care system, modifying and trying to improve it to the benefit of the local people, experiencing successes and failures, and little by little, advancing in their pursuit of better health care for everyone.

It is by learning from the experiences of such workers, by emulating and extending their efforts, modified to suit indigenous circumstances, that the way of revolution will slowly be mapped and the obstacles that lie in the pathway to health for all be overcome.

In order to surmount these obstacles, their nature must first be understood. In this chapter, and the two following, we shall look at the main problems that face the travellers on the revolutionary health care road, examine some possible solutions to these problems, and most importantly, report on some practical attempts at solutions that have been made in particular areas.

First, we shall look at the considerable difficulties that confront anyone attempting to achieve the full organizational and functional integration of hospital, primary health care, and other services.

Secondly, in Chapter 7, we shall discuss the changes required in the attitudes and orientation of all concerned with health care—givers and receivers alike—and the educational and training efforts that will be necessary to bring such changes about.

Thirdly, in Chapter 8, we shall consider the sort of information, finance and referral systems that the new style of health care system will demand.

Main problems

Coming then to the first set of problems, it is manifest that the integration of primary health care, hospitals and all the other services and agencies that comprise a successful comprehensive health system at national or local level, is easier said than done, and more easily done in some countries than others.

Like the WHO Expert Committee upon whose report (7) we draw so heavily throughout these chapters, we see the district health system as the appropriate setting in which to address and resolve these problems of integration.

Not unexpectedly, such problems are likely to be most easily solved in situations where all of the services necessary for the creation of a comprehensive district health system are not only available in one form or another but under the direct control of a single authority. Where different bodies—either separate governmental departments, or governmental and nongovernmental authorities—control different sections of the system, and where some sections may even be virtually non-existent, effective cohesion naturally becomes much more difficult.

As the Expert Committee pointed out, there are few countries where the government is solely responsible for the whole of the district health system. In most, to use the report's words "a mixture of government, social security, voluntary, private and industrial organizations comprise the health service". And, in such circumstances, "without effective coordination among all the agencies, the possibilities for unified or coordinated action to support primary health care at the district level are likely to be limited, and health priorities for the local population will be determined by the goals or interests of individual institutions" rather than "by the needs of the community" (7).

Even in situations where the district health system is under government control, it is usually, as the report suggests, "one sector within an overall social framework involving a number of government programmes", which "may be changed or expanded from time to time, not necessarily in step with each other", with the result that "programme management may be fragmented and scattered amongst different authorities, making it difficult to link all the programmes together so that they can make the most impact."

53

Then there are the inherent differences in the history, philosophy and style of the hospitals, primary health care and other services that constitute the district health system—differences that may well have already created wide disparities of practice and gaps in cooperation that will not easily be bridged.

As the report points out:

> Activity at the hospital level focuses on individual sophisticated technologies, and intensive treatment. It is often fast-paced, dramatic and short term. It requires professional control and dependence of the patient on the provider. Activity at primary health care level focuses on populations as well as individuals, and simple methods of treatment and prevention, and is generally slower in pace; people are required to be self-reliant and less dependent upon the providers. The traditional separation (and even antagonism) between the two types of activity forms an important barrier to functional coordination.

So, how is this barrier and the others that stem from differing philosophies of provision, different forms of

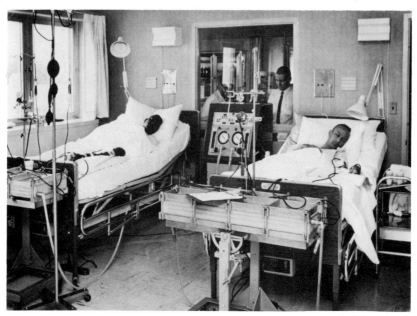

WHO Photo/NIH/E. Hubbard

"Activity at the hospital level focuses on individual sophisticated technologies . . ."

organization, a variety of administrative authorities, or simple gaps in service provision, to be overcome?

Overcoming the problems: approaches to solutions

First of all it is essential to get the facts straight—to know for example what sorts and qualities of health services are available at the district level, who provides them, what elements are missing, and what needs to be done to make the district health system both comprehensive and fully integrated.

Secondly, it is important to remember that the situation at district level will not only vary within countries but even more so between one country and another.

The WHO Expert Committee was in no doubt that "methods of analysing health systems should be developed in order to improve understanding of these [intercountry] differences and to help solve the problems of organizational and functional integration between hospitals and primary health care in different local situations."

The Committee felt that a broad, illustrative classification of different types of health system at the district level would be useful. Assessing the style and quality of district services in accordance with five criteria, therefore, it proposed that five main types of district health system could be distinguished.

Both the criteria and the five main types of system suggested by the Committee are listed below, with the classification also reproduced in tabular form.

The criteria were:

(i) the level of completeness of the referral arrangements and the extent of coordination between other services and the hospital;
(ii) the extent to which the population served by the district health service is specifically defined;
(iii) whether there is one or more than one hospital in the area;
(iv) the types of ownership of hospitals and other elements in the system; and
(v) the level of development of hospitals and other health care components, and the comprehensiveness of the services that they provide.

Five main types of system were suggested (Table 1).

(i) Systems with good coordination between the hospital and other local health services, and with well-defined boundaries.
(ii) Systems with less coordination and less clearly defined boundaries.

55

Table 1. Classification of district health systems

Type of health system	Subtypes	Examples	Needs for strengthening
I. Well-coordinated hospital and community care, with a well-defined boundary	Unified service of hospital and community care Parallel, but integrated, system of hospital and community care	China, Cuba, USSR Chile, Finland	Fuller integration
II. Less-coordinated hospital and community care, with less-defined boundary	*By governing body* PHC H 1. GO GO 2. GO NGO 3. NGO GO 4. NGO NGO 5. Various mixtures of 1–4 in the same country	Brazil, India (rural parts), Indonesia, Kenya	Links between hospitals and community services Definition of population served Coordination of different governing bodies
III. Less-coordinated systems with multiple hospitals and less-defined boundaries	*By governing body* PHC H 1. GO GO 2. GO NGO 3. NGO GO 4. NGO NGO 5. Various mixtures of 1–4 in the same country	Argentina, Japan, Mexico, Republic of Korea, USA, Western Europe (many parts)	Links between hospitals and community services Definition of population served Coordination of different governing bodies

IV. Developing systems with relatively weak primary health care	Some developing countries	Primary health care network
		Links between hospitals and community care
		Definition of population served (this may require the coordination of different governing bodies)
		Funding
V. Developing systems with relatively weak hospital	Some developing countries	Hospital services
		Links between hospitals and community care
		Definition of population served (this may require coordination of different governing bodies)
		Funding

PHC = Primary health care (community care); H = Hospital; GO = Government organization; NGO = Nongovernmental organization.

(iii) Systems with multiple hospitals, less coordination, and less clearly defined boundaries.

(iv) Systems in a developing stage with the other local health services being weaker than the hospital.

(v) Systems in a developing stage with hospitals that are weaker than the other local health services.

Reorienting district health systems

Armed with this sort of information, each country, the Committee suggested, might then set about reviewing its health system, looking particularly at the role of the hospital in relation to primary health care and its supporting infrastructure.

The results of such a review could be used as the basis for preparing options for reorienting the organization and functions of district health systems, taking into account issues of feasibility and effectiveness in relation to current political and socioeconomic situations.

An active programme for reorienting hospitals towards primary health care should consider changes to be made in organizational and functional inter-relationships, manpower development, management processes and governance, and community involvement.

Implementation of such a programme is not an easy task. It requires the support and involvement of the key components of the health service (which are not always forthcoming), strong leadership, and a high level of teamwork. An intensive political effort may also be needed to achieve consensus in the community, and to ensure that sufficient authority is given to the district level so that it can work effectively as a management unit.

In many instances, it may be best to implement the programme step by step, starting with a pilot or demonstration project. In this way it may be possible to reconcile potentially conflicting aspects of the programme and also educate the community into new styles of thinking and of action.

Examples of reorientation programmes

A number of countries have of course already experimented with such reorientation programmes and the Committee's report gave the following six examples of programmes designed to reorient hospitals towards primary health care.

(i) *Direct government involvement.* The government can be the main body for initiating the programme of reorientation when both the hospitals and other local health services are under its control. The programme can take one of two directions:

- total integration of the hospital into a unified district health care system under one management structure, or
- maintaining two parallel systems, and creating strong links between them to promote functional coordination and integration.

(ii) *Creation of a health council.* In situations where parts of the district health system are controlled by different government and nongovernmental bodies, a council could be created to coordinate all the health services and to stimulate other action to protect and promote the health of the whole population of the district.

The council would be likely to include representatives of the providers of hospital and other health services; the local community; government; insurance agencies; voluntary organizations; and other bodies that are active in health and related sectors in the defined area.

(iii) *Creation of a district health management team.* In similar situations to those described above, health professionals and managers from the community, as well as the hospital, could be appointed by central or local government, or other relevant authorities, to act as a management team to coordinate the hospital and other local health services in a defined area.

(iv) *"Contract" between hospital and other health care providers.* Another approach to reorientation in situations where the components of the district health system are controlled by a range of governing bodies is to make a "contract" (based on mutual agreement, and which may be informal) between the hospitals and other health care providers. Obviously, implementation of the contract cannot be automatically assumed, and some mechanism to monitor and enforce it is necessary. In some cases, contracts have served to protect the interests of the health care providers and not to promote the welfare of the community. Therefore the community should be a party to the contract.

(v) *Designation of a nongovernment hospital to coordinate primary health care.* In districts where government health services are weak or absent but a strong nongovernment hospital is present, that hospital should be encouraged to act as the first referral level and to help coordinate all the primary health care programmes in the district.

(vi) *Legislation and regulations.* Even in situations where the parts of the district health system are controlled by a mixture of governing bodies, an integrated health service can be created by introducing legislation and regulations to cover such matters as allocation of responsibilities, patterns of organization, and methods of coordinating functions between the different components of the system. Once the legislation and regulations are officially approved, the road to implementation is open. However, it is obviously important that such rules are formulated only after extensive analysis of the local situation, and are agreed upon by the various components of the health system, since only then are they likely to work.

Overcoming the problems: some practical examples

That necessity is the mother of invention is as true in the
health care field as any other. There can be no doubt, for
example, that much of the experimentation and change that
have taken place recently (and will continue to take place) in
the way that health care is provided to the people of the
world, has been inspired less by altruism than by rising costs
and economic recession.

But just as gales provide fruit to be gathered from under
the trees, so financial shortages act as a spur to the
achievement of more and, one hopes, better care more
cheaply.

Hence the current tendency in all industrialized countries to
treat patients outside the hospital ward whenever appropriate,
and for hospital stays to be kept to the shortest possible
time when admission cannot be avoided.

Hence, also, the acknowledgement by all countries of the
need to develop primary health care and to link it more
closely to supporting hospitals, so that a better, more
equitable health care system may result. Although in this
case—and especially in developing countries—the driving force
for change undoubtedly derives as much from compassion for
the people as from a desire for increased efficiency of service
provision.

If the second trend has yet to gather the sort of
momentum its supporters (including the authors of this book)
would like to see, this is undoubtedly due in part to inertia
and reaction but also, and perhaps largely, to the level of
health services already available across the world. In the
developed countries this level, despite current financial
difficulties, is still high enough to make the need for change
seem less urgent, and the case for better organization less
important, than they should be. In the developing countries,
on the other hand, both the need and the case for change
are manifest but, to use Dr Johnson's percipient phrase,
"poverty makes some virtues impracticable".[1]

Nevertheless, the number of instances of serious efforts
being made to improve health and wellbeing, by developing
primary health care services and creating close links and

---

[1] BOSWELL, J., *Life of Johnson*, Vol. IV.

liaisons between them and hospitals, is greater than one might think.

Five examples known to us were mentioned briefly in Chapter 5. A worldwide study of hospital involvement in primary health care in 105 countries, conducted by the International Hospital Federation from 1981 to 1983, reported 424 participating hospitals in 36 countries in all six WHO Regions, as being "deeply involved in primary health care activities" (2).

These are encouraging figures but as the Introduction to the report of the investigation suggests, they provide no cause for complacency. While the study showed that more hospitals were involved in primary health care than many people expected, it also showed that more hospitals could do more.

"Indeed", one might add, "much more". But leaving that aside and concentrating instead on the institutions that have done something worth reporting in this respect, the following examples of hospital-linked health care activity in the sphere of organizational and functional integration have, for the most part, been taken from papers prepared for the meeting of the WHO Expert Committee on the Role of Hospitals at the First Referral Level, referred to previously.

For the sake of continuity, the examples now presented are grouped under the same headings and taken in the same order as the list of "Examples of reorientation programmes" given on page 59.

Direct government involvement

A number of developed countries, including the Scandinavian nations, the USSR and the United Kingdom meet the criterion of having well integrated health care systems, mainly, if not exclusively, state-supported and directed. Most of these countries are now taking steps to develop and integrate primary health care services into their systems and to encourage more public participation in health matters. Progress, however, is relatively slow, although better in some countries than others. Finland and the United Kingdom are interesting examples.

In the United Kingdom, the system has been based on district health authorities since 1982, although the comprehensive nature of their responsibilities was somewhat reduced in 1985 by the reintroduction of separate Family Practitioner Committees to manage the family practitioner services—i.e., services provided by general medical practitioners, dentists, opticians, and chemists. This means that the local integration of health and social services now involves associations and joint meetings between three organizations—local authority social services departments, district health authorities, and family practitioner committees.

Attempts to extend community health services and involve the public more closely in health care provision through membership of health authorities, family practitioner committees and, particularly, community health councils, have so far met with some, as yet limited, success, although a number of major hospitals now have well established departments of community medicine.

Finland, on the other hand, is an example of a country where the development of primary health care seems to be progressing more rapidly, especially since the passing of the Primary Health Care Act of 1972.

The *raison d'être* for that Act appears to have been primarily financial. In the early 1970s Finnish health costs were growing almost twice as fast as the gross domestic product, apparently with no commensurate improvement in the health of the population.

But whatever the reason behind its introduction, the Act has certainly heralded an era in Finnish health provision when primary health care has become steadily more dominant. In the early 1970s 10% of health resources were devoted to it; today the figure is nearer 40%.

Every one of Finland's 461 communes (or local authorities) is now obliged by law to set up a health centre either on its own or jointly with its neighbours. These health centres are not single buildings but local organizations of health services, nearly all of which include local hospitals with beds mainly for observation, and the treatment of mild illnesses and chronic patients.

A considerable amount of rationalization is still necessary to improve the organization of services but, in any restructuring, primary health care will manifestly be well to the fore. In the words of an official publication on Finnish health services (*17*), the country's current health policy is based on "the promotion of healthy life habits, reduction of health hazards in the environment, and a slow but steady growth of services with prioritization of primary health care".

In this respect, Finland and China have something in common, for by Ministry of Health decree, all Chinese hospitals must contain a public health section.[1]

It is also noteworthy that in other countries, such as the United Republic of Tanzania and Yemen, primary health care units have been established at Ministry of Health level.[2]

Moving from national to local health services, mention has already been made (in Chapter 1) of the "hospital without walls" type of programme initiated and operated by the Carlos Luis Valverde Vega Hospital in Costa Rica and the Patan Hospital in Nepal.

Reports have also been received of similar kinds of experiments being successfully carried out by the United Christian Hospital in Hong Kong,[3] the Bethesda Tomohon Hospital in Indonesia,[4] and, in a more limited fashion, at the teaching hospital of the Makerere University Medical School of Uganda.[5]

More apposite to this particular discussion, however, is the Royal Southern Memorial Hospital in Melbourne, Australia, where the government—in this case of the State of Victoria—has cooperated with other local and national bodies (including the Australian Medical Association and the Royal Australian College of General Practitioners) to integrate hospital and other levels of care.

In the words of the hospital's Director of Community Care Services, "its founding philosophy . . . was to be a hospital without walls or an Open Hospital", and among its

---

[1] ZHENG, L. C. *The role of the commune hospital in primary health care.* Unpublished WHO document, SHS/EC/85/WP/III.A.6.

[2] AFRICAN MEDICAL AND RESEARCH FOUNDATION. *The role of the hospital at the first referral level: observations, comments, and some recommendations.* Unpublished WHO document, SHS/EC/85/WP/III.A.9.

[3] PATERSON, E. H. *First referral level hospital support for the community: a practitioner's view from Hong Kong.* Unpublished WHO document, SHS/EC/85/WP/III.C.2.

[4] SUPIT, B. A. *The first referral level hospital support for the local health system infrastructure (the Bethesda Tomohon Hospital involvement and experience, North Sulawesi, Indonesia).* Unpublished WHO document, SHS/EC/85/WP/II.D.1.

[5] NAMBOZE, J. *Community involvement at the first referral level hospital.* Unpublished WHO document, SHS/EC/85/WP/III.G.1.

essential aims were "to reintegrate general practitioners fully into the [hospital] staff structure", and "to provide integrated paramedical care and social support to the local community through referral by the family physician."

This concept of family medicine, based geographically and physically on the Community Care Centre built in the hospital in the early 1970s, has been highly successful. In 1969 there were 19 general practitioners affiliated to the Centre; by 1985 the number had grown to 160.[1]

Finally, it is relevant to make brief mention of three further reports of government action of a more parochial nature, which has nevertheless been taken in order to produce better integration of hospital and other health and allied services.

India, Kenya and Turkey are three countries where a local public official has been made specifically responsible for the integration of health care services in his/her district. Chief Medical Officers in India,[2] District Commissioners in Kenya,[3] and District Health Officers in Turkey[4] undertake this task.

As Professors Fisek and Erdal of the Haceteppe University of Ankara, Turkey, point out:[4]

> Primary health care programmes cannot be developed if the supervision of the service providers, starting with physicians in health centres and continuing to community health workers in the remote villages, is not carried out continuously and systematically. It is the most neglected activity in many developing countries.

Creation of a health council

Health councils or similar types of body exist in a number of countries.

The United Kingdom has its district health authorities together with (since the mid-1970s) joint planning and

---

[1] COMBES, J. B. *Experience in integrating levels of care from the concept of the 'Open Hospital.'* Unpublished WHO document, SHS/EC/WP/III.B.4.

[2] SAIGAL, M. D. *Organization and structural relationships of government, non-governmental and industrial first referral level hospitals in India.* Unpublished WHO document, SHS/EC/85/WP/III.ACE.1.

[3] OYOO, A. O. *First referral level hospital support for the local health system in Kenya.* Unpublished WHO document, SHS/EC/85/WP/III.A.2.

[4] FISEK, N. H. & ERDAL, R. *Hospital: an imperative for primary health care.* Unpublished WHO document, SHS/EC/85/WP/III.A.3.

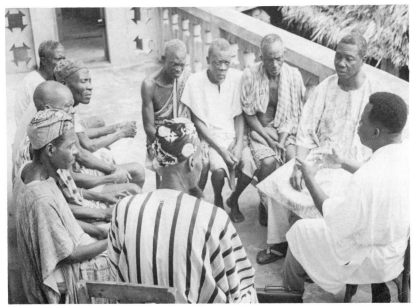

WHO Photo: P. Almasy

A village health council meeting.

financing committees with local authority social services departments—although as yet private health institutions are not included in any joint planning arrangements.

Finland has communal federations (too many in the view of its National Board of Health) for health centres, central and local general hospitals, mental hospitals and tuberculosis sanatoria.

In New South Wales, Australia, the Government established, in 1984, three experimental Area Health Boards to encompass all aspects of health, with the aim, after evaluation, of extending them throughout the State.[1]

Creation of a district health management team

District health management teams are not uncommon. They have existed in the United Kingdom since 1972—ten years

---

[1] AZMI, M. *Hospital support for the local health system in New South Wales.* Unpublished WHO document, SHS/EC/85/WP/III.A1.

prior to the creation of district health authorities—and other countries have also introduced them.

The District Health Management Teams in Kenya, for example, manifestly play a key role in the nation's health care system.[1] These nine-person teams of senior professional staff (Medical Officer of Health, Hospital Secretary, District Nursing Officer, District Public Health Officer, District Health Education Officer, District Public Health Nurse, District Nutrition Officer, District Clinical Officer, Pharmacist) function in both the hospital and the community and carry the responsibility for developing all local health care services. The teams are *directly* responsible *only* for government-provided services but one of their fourteen functions is "to liaise with non-government health organizations in the district".

In a paper on the Kasongo Public Health Project in Zaire[2]—a completely unified system of hospital and health centres—members of the Institute of Tropical Medicine of Antwerp, Belgium (which operates the project) also make special reference to a "direction team", which "organizes, supervises and coordinates all activities at all levels of the system," which provides health care to the 200 000 people of the Kasongo area.

For this most interesting project, which "promises to take responsibility for the health of the people in return for community participation in the running of the system and in health development", the direction team consists of the physicians of the 180-bed rural general hospital, its senior nursing staff and the administrator of the project.

"Contract" between hospital and other health care providers

The Kasongo Public Health Project also provides a practical example of a "contract" being made for the provision of health care services, although in this instance the

---

[1] OYOO, A. O. *First referral level hospital support for the local health system in Kenya.* Unpublished WHO document, SHS/EC/85/WP/III.A.2.

[2] DE BETHUNE, X. ET AL. *The role of the hospital in strengthening primary health care: the experience of Kasongo.* Unpublished WHO document, SHS/EC/85/WP/III.C.5.

"contractual arrangement" is between the providers and the public, rather than between a hospital and other providers. Even so, within the broadest definition of primary health care, the public, both from the points of view of being voluntary health workers and being self-helpers, *are* providers.

The aim of the contract is also wider than it first appears. As the writers of the Belgian paper say of the principles underlying the scheme:

It is expected that such a setting shall eventually enhance social consciousness and interest, as well as stimulate initiatives and innovations in other developmental fields. The final aim in this respect is to favour political decisions that would enhance equity and democracy.

Designation of a nongovernment hospital to coordinate primary health care

The provision and integration of hospital and primary health services by nongovernmental organizations, whether officially designated by governments or not, is commonplace in developing countries and even in some more developed areas—witness the work of the United Christian Hospital in Hong Kong, previously mentioned.

The Christian Medical Commission of the World Council of Churches has noted that in some countries "the church-related hospitals account for anywhere between 15% and 60% of medical and health care, and are situated in rural areas where they enjoy the confidence of the people they serve."

Many of these hospitals were pioneers of primary health care and now have community health departments and outreach programmes; they may assist with the local production of essential drugs, form links with traditional medical workers and define community health problems.

One such hospital—the Bethesda Tomohon Hospital in North Sulawesi, Indonesia—has divided itself into two sections, one of which deals *solely* with primary health care support activities. Equally in the Philippines, a number of community programmes linked to church hospitals operate successfully.

"We can learn from experiences in the Philippines and Indonesia" the Commission proposes "which have shown

67

that such programmes can be self-sustaining without excessive or continuous flow of outside capital."[1]

Other nongovernmental organizations, well known for their work in this sphere, include the African Medical and Research Foundation (AMREF) and the Aga Khan Foundation.

In its paper written for the WHO Expert Committee,[2] AMREF points out that many of the first referral level hospitals of East Africa are run by religious missions, and provide, in addition to curative services, networks of local dispensaries, mobile family planning and maternity and child health units (FP/MCH), and include in their outpatient services, programmes for health education, family planning, maternal and child health care, antenatal care, immunization and nutritional rehabilitation.

The Aga Khan Foundation has 110 health centres of varying kinds throughout the world, provides mobile "camps" for immunization and health education, and operates the new Aga Khan Hospital and Medical College which was recently built in Karachi—an institution designed to support primary health care in a variety of ways, and already granted university status by the Government.

Dr Tajuddin Manji, President of the Aga Khan Central Health Board for Pakistan (which is especially concerned with primary health care) believes that the Aga Khan Health Services "have an unprecedented opportunity, or more correctly an obligation, to create a working model of what may eventually become a truly comprehensive health care system" (6).

Legislation and regulations

Examples of the integration through legislation of hospital and primary health services provided by a variety of authorities are scanty.

A number of countries have created integrated health care systems as a consequence of legislation and central

---

[1] RAM, E. R. *Church-related hospitals: a first referral level experience.* Unpublished WHO document, SHS/EC/85/WP/III.C.3.

[2] AFRICAN MEDICAL AND RESEARCH FOUNDATION. *The role of the hospital at the first referral level: observations, comments and some recommendations.* Unpublished WHO document, SHS/EC/85/WP/III.A.9.

regulation. Among those that would claim to have done so could be included the USSR, the United Kingdom, Scandinavian nations, many other European countries and China.

In a number of these countries, private medical and paramedical services, including hospital care, are controlled, limited, or otherwise affected to some extent by legislation, partly for ideological reasons and partly to try to ensure the provision of the best possible health care to the people, while still retaining reasonable freedom of choice wherever possible, including choice between governmental and nongovernmental services.

Reference has also been made earlier to the Chinese Ministry of Health's decree that every hospital in the country must have a public health section, to the decisions taken in the United Republic of Tanzania and Yemen to establish primary health care units at ministry level, and to legislation in the Philippines which gave provincial hospitals overall responsibility for health care in their provinces.

Finally, Oyoo[1] has made reference to a policy decision taken by the Government of Kenya, which has undoubtedly affected the organization of health care locally. In July 1982 the Government introduced its "District Focus for Rural Development" strategy, whereby the responsibility for planning and implementing rural developments of all kinds, including developments in the health care field, was moved from the headquarters of ministries to the district level.

---

[1] See footnote 1, page 66.

Chapter 7. Problems of implementation: attitudes, orientation and training

Main problems

In its report, *Hospitals and health for all* (7), the WHO Expert Committee on the Role of Hospitals at the First Referral Level, listed half a dozen reasons—in addition to the more general ones of inertia, apathy, and reaction—why people throughout the world are likely to be resistant to or sceptical of the benefits of the health care revolution.

Members of the community may be ignorant of the local primary health care facilities, or they may mistrust them, either because the services are of unproven quality or because, like so many people, they have an over-glamourized view of hospitals.

The reasons may also be more mundane. In some countries where private medicine flourishes, hospitals may offer the only care and treatment that is either free or relatively inexpensive. It is also understandable that many sick people will go to the *nearest* point where health care is available, whatever sort of facility it happens to be, just as apprehension and distance may deter some people from going to hospital, and ignorance and indifference cause others to go nowhere at all.

As for those who work in hospitals, many tend to be too insular and isolationist in their attitudes to the other forms of health care provision that exist outside their institutions, and to regard them as of lesser quality than those with which they themselves are concerned.

70

There is a widespread tendency, in consequence, for community-based health staff to be less well rewarded than their hospital colleagues—both financially and in terms of social status—so that they are seen by the institutional workers as, and often feel themselves to be, inferior rather than equal partners in the battle for health.

As the WHO Expert Committee report says (7):

Hospitals are powerful, influential, and long-established—and hence intrinsically resistant to change. It is not enough simply to say that hospitals *should* change. Powerful levers and incentives will have to be used to make appropriate structural and administrative changes; to reorient job loyalty and responsibility towards health districts, and away from buildings and institutions; and to make parallel changes in the structure of training and teaching systems. Financial and status rewards can be powerful incentives for change, but in general support the *status quo*.

The way that many health care managers work typifies the Expert Committee's view. They are, as the Committee suggests, "usually more concerned with managing the existing hospital facilities adequately than with running the whole health system"—even though the savings inherent in an appropriate shift from hospital to primary health care are estimated by the Committee to be "as much as a third of total hospital costs".

In other words, if real advances are to be made towards better and more just health care systems, managers, like other leaders in the hospital field, will have to change, just as much as the rank and file of their health professional colleagues, and the institutions in which they work.

There is, indeed, a vicious circle, which creates reaction in hospital staff and which needs to be broken. Staff members see and feel themselves—and often rightly so—to be too heavily overburdened with work to extend their activities into primary health care even if they wanted to; a situation that certainly applies in the rural areas of many developing countries, as the investigation undertaken by the Royal Tropical Institute of Amsterdam demonstrates.[1]

The study was carried out by means of questionnaires sent to 70 hospitals in 14 countries in tropical Africa, where doctors who had previously been trained at the Institute were working.

---

[1] FOLMER, H. *Hospitals and primary health care*. Unpublished WHO document, SHS/EC/85/WP/III.A.8.

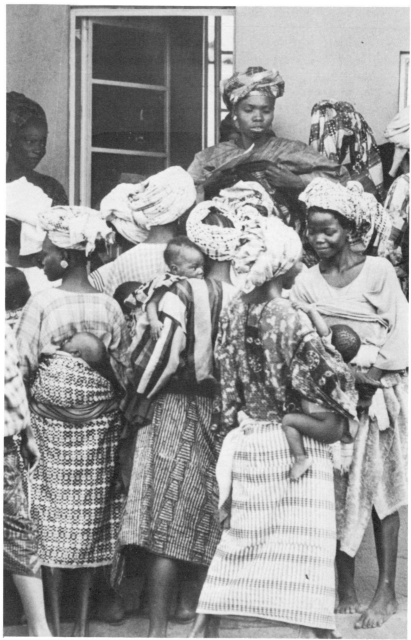

Overcrowding is a frequent problem in health facilities in developing countries.

The vast majority of those who replied saw themselves as becoming increasingly aware of the value of primary health care, and confirmed in many instances their participation in immunization activities and peripheral visits, but felt they were much too busy with hospital work to take on any more duties in the community.

It is a reaction and point of view, as the instigators of the survey wisely point out, that is as understandable as it is wrong:

> One can only conclude that by actively supporting all levels of health care below the hospital level, and thus helping to strengthen the quality and capacity of these levels, hospitals *can* break the vicious circle of their heavy workload.

But how are attitudes to be changed? The WHO Expert Committee had a number of suggestions to make which are worth repeating here.

Overcoming the problems: approaches to solutions

(a) *Changing attitudes.* Resistance to change can sometimes be a sign of inner strength, for instance in long-established hospitals, medical schools, and nursing schools. If this strength can be turned towards new purposes, for example, through strong leadership, then it can become a force *for* change, rather than against it. One approach that could be used to promote the interdependence of community and hospital services is to encourage respected peers or leaders to initiate change from within established institutions.

(b) *Redefining roles in service and education.* The hospital as an institution might benefit from being redefined as a community-health oriented institution, which means that it is not only disease-oriented but has responsibilities in the fields of preventive medicine and health promotion. It could then be used as a base for continuing education and training (professional, technical, and managerial) of community personnel. In this way the surrounding district can benefit from having highly-qualified staff who can provide advice at the community level, supervise community health auxiliaries, and contribute to their training.

(c) *Collecting data.* It is important that increased back-up from hospitals for community health professionals and auxiliaries should serve to meet the real needs of the community. In this respect it is vital that field workers have the training and ability to collect and transmit appropriate data to the relevant levels of the health system, whether it be simple information on household health and socioeconomic conditions, or more complicated epidemiological and technical data. In time, collection and analysis of essential data should become routine. Such information can radically broaden people's awareness and change their values by showing them needs of which they were previously unaware. It can thus promote changes in attitudes and in services.

(d) *Emphasis on community health in training.* The increased emphasis on community health should be reflected in the training of health workers, both in terms of curriculum content and the site of training—with trainers and students based for at least 20–25% of their time in primary health care settings. Training institutions should select their trainees not only for their scientific and technical abilities but also for their commitment to the welfare of people; in some cases commitment to primary health care should be the most important criterion for selection. Health personnel involved in primary health care must have a sensitive approach to social and emotional problems and thus training programmes should aim to develop psychosocial skills; they should also develop the skills that enable people to work as part of an effective team. Since initial training may not immediately be used in the primary health care context, it is important that mechanisms for continuing education be established that repeatedly reassert the principles of community-oriented practice.

(e) *Modification of teaching structures.* In existing systems it is usually the case that teachers and lecturers (for example, in medical faculties) are appointed to universities (or other institutions) that have a clinical base in a hospital. It is worth considering whether such an attachment could be to an entire health district, with teaching and clinical responsibility to the district, not merely to a hospital.

(f) *Defining effectiveness.* It is just as important for training schools and health administrations to help to define appropriate indicators of performance in primary health care, as it is for health agencies and administrations to define precisely the tasks that are required to meet the health needs of the population. Performance indicators concerned with whether a hospital has become an effective part of a district health system are particularly important. However, the Expert Committee recognized that it is more difficult to define effectiveness in the field of primary health care than in the traditional curative sector.

(g) *Collaboration in training.* In places where training resources are scarce, it may be necessary and desirable to encourage several institutions to collaborate in primary health care training, for example, by inviting visiting professors from other universities and from business and management schools, and by arranging joint courses, multidisciplinary field practice, etc. Sometimes, it may be useful to share experiences with universities and any other training institutions that are innovative in the field of primary health care training programmes, including institutions that are willing to introduce such programmes but do not know how to do so. WHO may be able to play an important role in promoting such an exchange of information. WHO might also help by designating certain training centres or health districts as collaborating centres in integrated health care.

In addition, national hospital associations and/or associations of hospital and health services managers can play a major role in helping to improve standards of management and management training.

(h) *Incentives to change.* None of the training processes will meet the objective of better integration of preventive and curative services within the district health system if there is no explicit incentive to change. It is therefore necessary for countries to consider, as a priority, the need to improve both the status and the financial rewards for those working in community-oriented services so that differences between hospital and community personnel, in these respects, are lessened. If key senior professionals who now work in hospitals were to work part-time in community settings, it would improve the social standing of personnel who are community trained and oriented, and enhance integration in training and service. Similarly, people in management and leadership positions need to be able to take a broad view of health needs, and of ways in which (within resource constraints) they can be better met. Among other things, this may call for changes in the recruitment of managers and in their training, terms of appointment, and performance appraisal.

The Expert Committee emphasized that social change is a long-term process that cannot be achieved by hasty or premature evaluation of education and training policies and programmes.

That final comment is an important one, and prompts us to reiterate our previously expressed view that the health care revolution is a reformation that will take time to achieve. Nevertheless, in the area of revolution concerned with changing the attitudes and overcoming the prejudices of people, work has already been done, ideas put into practice, and some advances made. The following practical examples of activities in this sphere are mainly culled from papers presented to the WHO Expert Committee, and are presented serially in accordance with the "approaches to solutions" listed above.

Overcoming the problems: some practical examples

Changing attitudes

Mention has already been made of several hospitals in different countries where, with the support of senior staff, a policy of active liaison with primary health care services has been implemented. These include the Carlos Luis Valverde Vega Hospital, San Ramón, Alajuela, Costa Rica; the Patan Hospital, Kathmandu, Nepal; the Royal Southern Memorial Hospital in Melbourne, Australia; and the United Christian Hospital, Kwun Tong, Hong Kong.

Similarly, we have referred to the extramural activities in the community being carried out by the Department of Paediatrics, Makerere University Medical School, Uganda.

Reports from China have also stressed the importance placed there on leading health care officials being seen to support primary health care.[1,2] The Chinese believe that "all

---

[1] ZHENG, L.-C. *The role of the commune hospital in primary health care.* Unpublished WHO document, SHS/EC/85/WP/III.A.6.

[2] CHEN LONG. *The three-level medical and health care network in rural areas, and the role of county-level institutions in primary health care.* Unpublished WHO document, SHS/EC/85/WP/III.A.10.

administrative and political leaders, especially the directors of the health departments at each level of care, should pay great attention to primary health care, and always keep it in mind, write about it and implement it in action."

Finally, it is worth noting that in the Kasongo Public Health Project in Zaire, part of the implementation strategy involved maximum delegation of clinical responsibility to nurses. They assumed, as the report puts it, "tasks . . . as complex as meningitis or tetanus diagnosis and treatment, or surgical procedures," which meant "that the role of the physician changed . . . and for all standardisable tasks . . . became one of support and counselling, rather than . . . therapist."

This is an important development even though it may appear to stress the nurse's role in the hospital (albeit the first referral level hospital) rather than in the community.

For, as the Kasongo report emphasizes, it also enhances the status of nurses as a professional group in the eyes of the people, and the nurse's role "as a major provider of primary health care requires no major extension of a function that is already implicit in the definition of nursing."

The words are those of the International Council of Nurses, and the report from which they come[1] makes crystal clear just how much of a major source of health care nurses are. According to the latest global data, there are currently over four million professional nurses and eight million auxiliary nurses.

Redefining roles in service and education

The hospitals referred to above are already fulfilling the role of "community health oriented institutions" as envisaged by the WHO Expert Committee. Another, undertaking similar functions, is the Nangina Mission Hospital in Kenya, a 78-bed institution serving a local population of 55 000 as well as people from across the border in neighbouring Uganda.

---

[1] INTERNATIONAL COUNCIL OF NURSES. *Nursing care in the community and at the first referral level.* Unpublished WHO document, SHS/EC/85/WP/II.D.2.

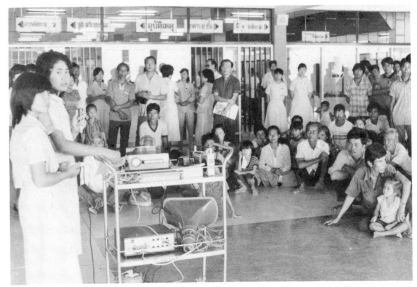

WHO Photo: J. Ling

Health education of the community in a provincial hospital.

Nangina Hospital, like the other mission hospitals in Kenya, seems to be an example of a hospital virtually designated by the government to provide integrated care in its local area.

The trend towards community health oriented hospitals can also be seen in other countries. Hungary, for example, is moving towards an extension of its hospital-polyclinics to form territorial Patient Care Units, "in the framework of which all primary health care services in the catchment area would be included in the organizational unit of the hospital-polyclinic."[1]

A similar development is a longer-term objective both in India, where the aim is to develop community health centres that would function as first level referral hospitals, and in Finland where instead of expecting "to receive patients who either walk in or are transported in . . . the hospital should

---

[1] SITKERY, I. *First referral level hospital support for the local health system in Hungary.* Unpublished WHO document, SHS/EC/85/WP/III.A.4.

influence the incidence and prevalence of disease and the activities of care in the field."

The way forward to community health oriented hospitals is not always easy to follow. Interestingly enough, one of the earliest and best known examples of such a hospital—the Carlos Luis Valverde Vega Hospital in Costa Rica—has been fighting for a decade to retain its 'hospital without walls' programme. The central authority in the country, for reasons of its own, would prefer to see the hospital returned to exclusively or largely curative activities, a course of action opposed by the local people, who are prepared to battle for what they see as their right to have a say in the way that health care is provided in their area.

It is a spirit to be admired for it would indeed be sad if what an eminent Latin American social scientist has called "the little bird of public participation in health—very pretty but very fragile", should find itself destroyed by controversy.

Collecting data

In the investigation of 70 hospitals in 14 tropical African countries, undertaken a few years ago by the Royal Tropical Institute of Amsterdam to discover the extent of their primary health care liaison, only a minority of respondents—18 or 40%—reported that they collected village level data, and even fewer—6 or 13%—gave any information on how the data were used.

The importance of adequate and relevant information to an effective health care system at any level is self-evident, and is stressed in two papers presented to the WHO Expert Committee which give advice in some detail on what sort of data are needed in the primary health care sphere and how best the information may be collected and used.[1, 2]

Examples of data actually collected, however, are not plentiful. The WHO Collaborating Centre for Primary Health

---

[1] SUBRAMANIAN, M. *Information systems support to first referral level hospitals in developing countries: an example.* Unpublished WHO document, SHS/EC/85/WP/II.A.3.
[2] LEWIS, C. A. *Design and use of health records in the local health system.* Unpublished WHO document, SHS/EC/85/WP/II.A.4.

Care in Jiading County, Shanghai, China, reports that rural doctors in the country maintain simple records at village health stations (patient visits, immunization, births, deaths) and provide quarterly data on medical services, epidemic prevention, and maternal and child health care, as well as an annual summary report, to the township health centres.

A more detailed system is in operation in Manila, Philippines, where over a quarter of the 899 *barangays* which comprise the city, are officially designated as depressed or disadvantaged areas. A *barangay*, or neighbourhood, is the lowest political unit of government in the country and the 248 depressed ones in Manila have a collective population of over half a million—30% of the total for the city.

As part of a scheme to improve general health and social standards in these areas, *barangay* health volunteers are undertaking the vital task of collecting data. In 1984 a Family Sheet was introduced as a tool to help develop the Health Information Monitoring System. The Family Sheets are distributed and collected by a health centre nurse every three months and are completed by families as part of a day-to-day routine. Information included in the sheet covers the family profile, its living conditions, sanitation, livelihood, assets and income, and data on simple complaints (pain, fever, coughs, colds, diarrhoea, etc.) for each family member. The health sheets reflect the trend of minor health problems in the area and provide a survey of the utilization of health services.[1]

The work being done in Manila is a more advanced form of the sort of local data collection undertaken in some countries under the general heading of "community mapping", whereby, as both a training method and a diagnostic tool for primary health care development, voluntary health workers collect details during home visits of the prevailing health problems of a community and record them in symbols on a rough map of the locality. (See, for example, the report on the SSA Hospital in the city of Netzacualcoyotyl, Mexico, by Macagba (2).)

---

[1] SUNA, E. G. *A lay reporting mechanism for the development of a health information monitoring system in urban primary health care—the Manila experience.* Unpublished WHO document, DES/LR/HFA/85.4.

79

Emphasis on community health in training and modification of teaching structures

Community nurses and community physicians are trained in a number of industrialized countries. Examples of hospital-supported training can be found in many countries and territories including Australia, Hong Kong, Kenya, Lesotho, Nepal and Turkey.

The United Christian Hospital in Hong Kong, for example, started training community nurses before the new hospital was built, and also uses student nurses as visiting Family Health Advocates.

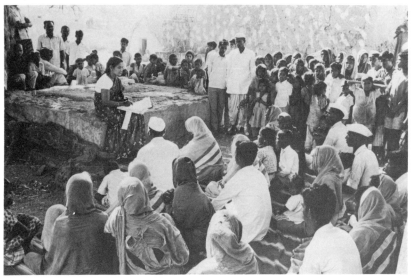

Photo: WHO/UN

Health education in the community.

In *Hospitals and primary health care* (2), details are given of educational and training programmes designed to improve primary health care at, *inter alia*, The Lady Hardinge Medical College and associated hospitals in New Delhi, India, the Wad Medani Civil Hospital in Medani, Sudan, the Ramathibodi Hospital in Bangkok, Thailand, and the Soroka Medical Centre in Beer Sheva, Israel.

At the last-mentioned, selection of medical students is refreshingly linked to the health—and human—needs of people:

Fifty students are admitted annually to the first year class. Before admission the student is interviewed by a committee that includes ten physicians and ten laymen from the community. Community orientation is looked for in attitude, behaviour and experience of the applicant. Empathy is valued along with the ability to communicate with people from various social backgrounds. Motivation to work within a developing community is essential.

A similar attitude is exemplified in the way that the Aga Khan Health Services select and train their various primary health care workers (6):

As important as where we provide our services is how these services are provided. In a developing country it is not enough just to have primary care centers. People have to be made aware of how to fully utilize the facilities available. A personal relationship of confidence and trust must be developed between the people and the local health worker. Over the years, the Aga Khan Central Health Board has developed an extensive system of selection and training—identifying qualified people at the local level and moving them through a training progression as they demonstrate their interests and capabilities. A worker may begin as an assistant mid-wife, advance to a mid-wife, and eventually progress to a lady health visitor position—the key person in our primary health care system.

It is a selection and training process of which the International Council of Nurses would approve, for as it quite rightly complains:[1]

The majority of basic nursing education programmes in most countries continue to be operated in hospitals, by hospitals and for hospitals—and they are primarily procedure-oriented, with little or no orientation to the community.

This is despite the fact that community health nurses, as the Council points out, can play a vital role in community health education, in training primary health care workers,

---

[1] INTERNATIONAL COUNCIL OF NURSES. *Nursing care in the community and at first referral level.* Unpublished WHO document, SHS/EC/85/WP/II.D.2.

planning and evaluating primary health care programmes, supervising community health workers, and in liaison between first referral level hospitals and peripheral health units.

Defining effectiveness

It is not always easy to produce performance indicators in the health care field that are of real value in assessing the effectiveness of health services, rather than being merely quantitative measures of health activities. In the area of hospitals, experience in a number of countries, including the United States of America and the United Kingdom has already demonstrated this. The primary health care reviews conducted in several developing countries with the aid of WHO have usually not looked into the hospital involvement in primary health care. The investigation by questionnaire carried out by the Royal Tropical Institute of Amsterdam, (see page 71) is a step towards clarification of the interaction.

The designers of the Royal Tropical Institute's study concluded, for example, that using the information gathered from the replies to its questionnaires:

> It should be possible to construct a 'PHC-support index' with which the involvement of a hospital can be measured or expressed in quantitative terms. Such an index, however, would have to take into account not only the quantified activities in primary health care, but also the hospital's size, staff and curative workload.

Its recommendations to others wishing to try to define effectiveness of primary health care support by hospitals, however, included the following advice:

> The inventory should be extended to other continents [in addition to Africa] and another method, preferably using on-the-spot visits to a larger sample of hospitals.

Collaboration in training and incentives to change

Specific examples of interinstitutional training for primary health care workers are hard to find, as are examples of deliberate attempts to improve the rewards and status of such workers.

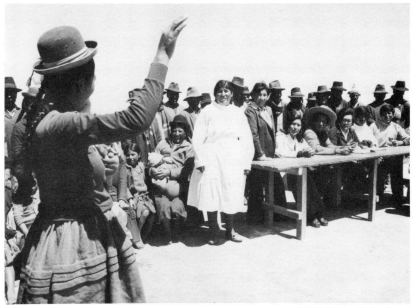

WHO Photo: Y. Pouliquen

It is important that members of the community should be involved in decisions affecting their health.

However, examples can be quoted of a number of hospitals—from large teaching institutions to small rural hospitals—that are particularly oriented to the support of primary health care and the teaching of its staff.

The Soroka Medical Centre at Beer Sheva, Israel, is one such teaching institution and the Aga Khan Medical College and Hospital in Karachi is another. The Nangina Hospital, Samia, Kenya, also sends hospital staff to visit communities, supervise trainers, interview trainees and generally monitor training programmes, as well as to conduct mobile clinics.

In Turkey, preservice and in-service training is given by local hospital staff to their health centre colleagues, and in western Uganda one local hospital sends its staff—medical and other—into the catchment area to train primary health care workers, see referred cases, carry out immunizations, and visit self-help projects.

In the USSR and Hungary, it is common for specialists to make regular visits to remote areas, particularly in connection with obstetric, gynaecological, and paediatric services.

Many other nations could undoubtedly quote similar activities.

Chapter 8. Problems of implementation: information, financing and referral systems

Complex ventures require good organization if they are to succeed. In this respect the WHO Health for All programme is no different from any other task of similar magnitude. The sort of comprehensive health system that it proposes— provided partly *by* the people as well as *to* them, matched to their needs, community-oriented and district-based—will only operate successfully if it is efficiently organized.

As a WHO Expert Committee put it more tersely (7): "An integrated health system demands the integration of management techniques."

In this chapter we shall look at three subsystems of the general management system, i.e., information systems, financial arrangements and referral systems, at the problems of implementing them effectively in a comprehensive district health service, and at some possible solutions to these problems.

Once again, as in Chapters 6 and 7, reference is made to the views expressed by the WHO Expert Committee on the Role of Hospitals at the First Referral Level on these aspects of a remodelled health service.

Information systems

It is evident that all organizations, in every field of activity, require adequate and appropriate information if they are to operate effectively. Health services are no exception to this, and the sort of district system based on primary health care that we wish to see introduced worldwide will require regular and accurate data. Such data must provide details of both the tasks to be accomplished and the resources available, and must include information on the population to be served and its health needs, the extent and quality of the resources available to meet those needs, and regular reports on the efficacy with which the resources are used.

Main problems

The Expert Committee was of the opinion that, in general, health care information systems collect too little data on the way of life of the population to be served—on the households and families of which it is comprised, on the health and ailments of the individuals, and on the health hazards of their environment.

In addition, the Committee believed that such systems often work less well than they should because they suffer from various faults and deficiencies (7). Too many health care systems, it suggested:

- are hospital- or clinic-oriented rather than people-oriented;
- do not cover the most needy groups;
- are underutilized;
- try to collect too much data, mainly for centralized decision-makers;
- need highly-qualified people to obtain or interpret data;
- present numerical information without comparative data;
- give incorrect information because of the use of inappropriate methodologies and/or inadequate training and supervision of information gatherers;
- collect data about inputs and activities rather than health status and outcomes;
- fail to analyse information sufficiently; and
- fail to feed back analysed information to the community and to health care workers.

Manifestly, however, not all information systems in all countries are defective, and in some of those that have less than adequate arrangements, steps are being taken to remedy deficiencies. The United Kingdom, for example, is currently much concerned with improving the way in which information about the working of its National Health Service is collected and used.

86

Overcoming the problems: approaches to solutions

In the Expert Committee's view, the search for such improvement can be made easier if certain broad guidelines are followed (7). While it did not mention any country by name, it nevertheless noted that:

Practical experience from a number of countries that have developed effective information systems indicates the importance of:

– designing a system that enables simple home-based information to be collected by appropriately-trained community health workers (under professional supervision) in defined geographical neighbourhoods of 100–150 households;
– bringing this information together at different levels of the district health service and combining it with more detailed and sophisticated data relevant to health posts/centres and hospitals at the first referral level;
– organizing the system so that at each level the data-gathering and reporting mechanisms focus solely on information that (i) should be shared with people, (ii) is needed at each health care level, and (iii) needs to be passed on to other relevant decision-making levels; and
– presenting the results in a form that will facilitate decisions on adjustments in content and emphasis of current programmes, and on the need for new programmes and reallocation of resources.

The Expert Committee also made clear its belief that, in the pursuit of an effective community-oriented information system, the hospital at the first referral level has a key role to play. Appropriate activity on its part, it suggested, can be of great benefit to both the health district and the hospital itself.

The hospital at the first referral level can be encouraged to help in promoting a community-oriented information system by enlisting its assistance in:

– devising survey procedures;
– designing forms, questionnaires, and report sheets;
– training community health workers and other field staff;
– orienting doctors, nurses, and other health professionals;
– providing logistic support (for example, photocopying facilities, provision of forms, etc.); and
– analysing and evaluating data and providing feed-back to the community.

The potential benefits of a community-based information system for the hospital at the first referral level include:

– helping the hospital to identify more accurately the true needs of the population it serves;
– helping it to make decisions on what services need to be expanded or reduced (or added or discontinued), and on what kinds of assistance to give to health posts/centres linked to it;

- helping it to define community needs that could be met by intersectoral collaboration; and
- helping it to develop a more effective referral system, which could lead to a reduction of the hospital's workload by screening out patients who could be satisfactorily treated at health posts or health centres.

Overcoming the problems: some practical examples

A number of practical examples of relevance to a consideration of information systems have already been given in Chapter 7.

Mention was made there of the survey of hospitals in tropical Africa undertaken by the Royal Tropical Institute of Amsterdam, of the report from the WHO Collaborating Centre for Primary Health Care in Jiading County in China, of the introduction of Family Health Sheets in Manila, Philippines, and of community mapping in Mexico and elsewhere.

A brief reference was also made in that section, to two papers presented at the Expert Committee meeting, which are particularly concerned with the theory of collection and analysis of health information, and although it may seem at first sight somewhat paradoxical to speak of theory in a section concerned with practical examples, some of the advice given in those papers merits reproduction here because of its practical value.

The paper, *Information systems support to first referral level hospitals in developing countries*, for example, reminds us that such hospitals must collect information not only to help the development of primary health care services but also for their own direct needs and for higher echelons of the health care system.[1]

In a good health service the inter-relationships between the various levels of care should be clear and close-knit, and as the paper states:

Information available at the first referral level hospitals about peripheral primary health care services are used at that level not only to control, guide and support the primary health care services but also for adjusting the services provided by the first referral level hospitals themselves.

---

[1] Unpublished WHO document, SHS/EC/85/WP/II.A.3(a).

In order to collect information, it is necessary, of course, to decide what should be collected and how, and in these respects the paper *Design and use of health records in the local health system*, prepared by C. A. Lewis, President of the International Federation of Health Records Organizations, is most helpful.[1]

It suggests that three types of health records are necessary in primary health care—family, community and individual.

> Family health records are generally maintained in areas where household visits are part of the primary care services offered . . . The community 'health record' is a composite of numeric data (e.g. age and sex distribution of the population, number of births per year, number of deaths by selected age groups and cause, immunization levels, per cent of dwellings with adequate disposal of excreta, number of health workers by type); narrative data (e.g. major health problems, community organization, community leaders); and diagrams.

Individual health records, of course, are personal reports giving details of a particular subject and of his or her illnesses, and are used at the home, health centre and hospital.

Because different countries have different sorts of health workers of varying levels of education, training and experience, and a variety of approaches to the provision of services and their priority, it is essential that each develops its own primary health care case records, benefiting whenever possible from the experience of others.

The steps to be followed in designing the record, however, are the same for all:

- define the purpose the record must serve,
- describe the health care system,
- define the activities to be performed and by whom,
- define the procedure for these activities,
- define the reporting and recording requirements,
- select the most appropriate terminology, and
- design the form and test it before bringing it into use.

There is also much to be said for the standardization of record forms at the national level, even though different

---

[1] Unpublished WHO document, SHS/EC/85/WP/II.A.4.

versions of standardized forms may be required in, for
example, health centres and hospitals. In at least one
country, as the paper points out, "the process of designing
the [standard] form led to the establishment of the
standards of care".

Finally, case records and patient referral systems are
naturally closely interlinked, a point that we shall consider
in more detail later in this chapter.

Financing systems

The effects of rising costs and economic recession on health
services throughout the world were mentioned in Chapter 7.
They have produced obvious and considerable financial
difficulties in most countries, especially where they have
coincided with a national policy of trying to reallocate
health resources more evenly throughout the population.
They have also been responsible in some areas for the
achievement of improvements in the organization and
provision of services, as managers, planners, and clinicians
have risen to the challenge of trying to do more with less.

"We have no money, so we must think"—a comment
originally made by the distinguished scientist Lord
Rutherford—has been the watchword, during the past
decade, of many a health worker contemplating a much
desired new development with everything to commend it but
its cost. And now this eminently quotable phrase is once
again most apt, as we consider ways and means of
increasing and extending primary health care services during
this period of worldwide economic retrenchment.

Main problems

In the WHO Expert Committee's opinion, "ways must be
considered of generating the resources needed to support
increased hospital participation in primary health care and
of overcoming the barriers that block attempts to utilize
resources for this purpose."

These barriers will take some moving and those whose
task it is to organize such removal will be faced at every
level of the health care pyramid with the most difficult
decisions.

90

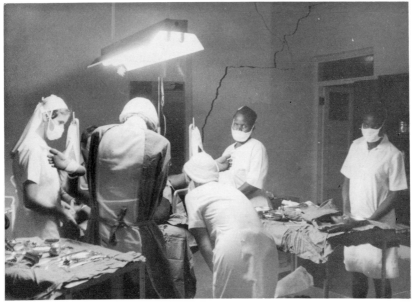

WHO Photo: R. Crow

It needs to be remembered that facilities will require regular maintenance.

Governments, for example, will have to weigh the pros and cons of giving the health sector a greater slice of the national economic cake, to the possible detriment of other sectors such as housing, education or defence.

Health authorities will be called on to look again at the knotty problems of equitable financial allocation. The hospital sector has traditionally received the lion's share of available health care funds. Moreover, within that sector, the larger urban hospitals have commonly been favoured at the expense of peripheral district hospitals.

Hospital clinicians—especially consultant doctors in the more esoteric specialities—will have to consider yet again whether they can continue to try to offer optimal treatment to their particular patients when others, less dramatically ill perhaps, are likely to be denied even a reasonable standard of care in the community.

Managers will have to face up to the similarly awkward implications of the "manager–patient relationship", and try

91

to the best of their ability to ensure that, as far as is humanly possible, all patients at every level of care, receive the best deal that limited resources can buy.

Despite the complexity of the problems, the WHO Expert Committee had views on how they might be overcome, and it is well worthwhile to reproduce them here.

Overcoming the problems: approaches to solutions

(i) *A dialogue among key participants in the health service.* One way of strengthening financial support for involvement in primary health care is to develop a dialogue among administrators of hospitals and other local health services, health professionals, third-party payers (employers, insurance companies, etc.), and government policy makers. Together they can explore ways of tapping unused or underused resources, inside and outside the district, and decide how to respond to unmet needs, especially of deprived population groups. Mutual understanding of the perspectives and priorities of each sector of the health service is essential for such an approach to succeed, as is community involvement in order to define priorities clearly.

(ii) *Flexibility in financing.* As a result of the kind of dialogue described above, key administrators may decide to make the budgets of hospitals under their jurisdiction more flexible in order to promote active participation in primary health care. They may even insist that a proportion of the budget be spent on primary health care programmes, or give financial incentives to encourage hospitals to become integrated into district services (for example, by giving more money to those hospitals that are committed to primary health care). Alternatively, they could decide to provide funds to a district health system rather than separately to hospitals and other services.

In some countries, ways of encouraging people and communities to contribute towards the cost of care, in terms of both financial and non-financial support, have been explored. One option is the use of civic groups, volunteer health workers, and health assistants for specific primary health care activities. Another may be the participation of families in caring for, and even providing food for, their hospitalized relatives.

(iii) *Appropriate financial and management information systems.* A task force, with representatives from various components of the district health system, could design, test, and refine a comprehensive financial and management information system that would help decision-makers allocate funds for specific needs and priorities. The system could include performance indicators so that cost-effectiveness could be assessed. The task force could invite people from within the health service, or outside it, to help design the system. It could also decide how to obtain the understanding and acceptance needed to make the system work, and how to train people to use it. The task force could formulate programmes for basic and continuing education and training of managerial and financial staff, and could also consider how to orient health professionals towards cost-control and cost-effectiveness.

(iv) *Making the system work.* Unless the results of financial and management reporting systems are used properly, such systems are worthless. Mechanisms need to be instituted that will bring together key people within the district health system to review and discuss the reports provided by the information system and their own observations and perceptions of needs and problems. Representatives from the different levels of the health service, consumers, politicians and other key figures could be included in these discussions. The objectives of the participants should be to agree on:

- issues or priority needs that demand changes or adjustments;
- what those changes should be; and
- who should implement them.

Overcoming the problems: some practical examples

The first point that needs to be made in any commentary on finance and primary health care is that primary health care facilities will not necessarily be inexpensive; a community-based service will not automatically be cheaper than the hospital equivalent it replaces.

In this connection the comments of the Christian Medical Commission, quoted in Chapter 6, will bear quoting again at greater length.

Under the subheading *Financing of primary health care*[1] the following views are expressed:

Recent studies have shown that many primary health programmes are not cheap and have not become self-reliant as rapidly as we expected. In certain cases the difficulty can be traced back to an excessive capital outlay at the initiation of the programme. This has often led to the instalment of physical facilities and the employment of personnel, making high demands on running costs. In many instances, primary health care programmes were started on a large scale and expanded too quickly.

Yet we can learn from experiences in the Philippines and Indonesia which have shown that such programmes can be self-sustaining without excessive or continuous flow of outside capital. Thus, in the long run, the most significant source of finance resides in the creation of new health resources from within local communities themselves. Their success seems to depend on the development of credit cooperatives, farming, fishing and industrial cooperatives and health insurance schemes.

Consideration should be accorded to community participation in community services. In most communities (including many in Asia, Africa and Latin America) financing is likely to be a combined effort between the community, the church hospitals and the government. Individual payment on a fee-for-service basis should be encouraged. The external financial support required by many hospitals for immediate use could be used to initiate primary health care programmes and to stimulate local appropriation. However, care should be taken that external financing does not replace local efforts, which are needed to ensure the continuity and further development of primary health care.

---

[1] RAM, E. R. *Church-related hospitals: a first referral level experience.* Unpublished WHO document, SHS/EC/85/WP/III.C.3.

The general tenor of these opinions is supported in a paper from the Institute of Public Health in Kampala, Uganda,[1] where a similar comment is made on how the members of the community can help to meet the costs of primary health care services.

> Besides contributing funds, the community can contribute labour, materials and expertise . . . Indigenous technology can be applied more easily if the community identifies itself with the hospital.

The development of primary health care can also be financed from other levels of service provision—national and regional, as well as local.

In some countries extension is being brought about by central policy decisions taken by the government, often in the form of periodic socioeconomic plans in which primary health care is given priority over further hospital or other development.

Finland, as has previously been demonstrated, is a prime example of this approach: Hungary, India, the USSR, and to a lesser extent, Guinea, are others, and there are many more. The same sort of policy, but implemented at a lower organizational level, is exemplified by the creation and terms of reference of the Area Health Boards of New South Wales, Australia, and the Direction Team of the Kasongo Public Health Project in Zaire.

And, to conclude this brief list of practical examples, it is apposite to remind readers that any financial intervention that causes hospitals to be more economic in their use of funds could be of benefit to the expansion of primary health care services.

In this connection, the introduction of Diagnosis Related Group payment mechanisms in the hospitals of the United States of America and elsewhere, and the experiments with clinical budgeting currently under way in the United Kingdom, are both worthy of note.

Referral systems

As we suggested in the first section of this chapter, records and referral systems are closely interlinked. Continuity of

---

[1] NAMBOZE, J. M. *Community involvement at the first referral level hospital.* Unpublished WHO document SHS/EC/85/WP/III.G.1.

patient care, especially in a multi-level health system, depends on both systems being well designed and operated.

A paper from the International Federation of Health Records Organizations (see page 89) lists 11 important ways in which health records staff can help to improve the referral process, from reviewing record data and appointments arrangements, to checking referral notes passing between levels of care, monitoring health centre and community worker referral rates, and hospital clinic revisit rates.

These forms of assistance are set in apposition to a list of some thirteen problems that are likely to occur in the referral process: problems that range from unnecessary referrals by health workers to hospitals, failures to refer when appropriate and incorrect self-referrals, to lack of knowledge or mistrust of community health services on the part of hospital staff and—that universal difficulty—failure by the hospital staff to provide adequate discharge information to their primary health care colleagues.

This same paper quotes the steps in the referral process defined by Williams et al. (*18*) a quarter of a century ago:

(i) Definition of need for and purpose of the referral; mutual understanding about these between referring physician and patient.
(ii) Adequate communication of this purpose and of problems for which help is needed.
(iii) Attention given to these needs and problems by the consultant.
(iv) Adequate communication of consultant's findings and recommendation to referring physician.
(v) Clear understanding by patient, referring physician and consultant of responsibility for the patient's continuing care.

This outline was obviously produced by doctors working in a developed country but, allowing for that, it is applicable, in principle, to the same process in any country.

The WHO Expert Committee, however, based its considerations of the problems of referral systems on a broader and perhaps less precise concept, which includes "not only the two-way referral of individual patients but also other forms of two-way consultation and support".

Main problems

In this context the Committee divided the difficulties inherent in organizing an efficient referral system into four key problems of patient referral, as follows:

95

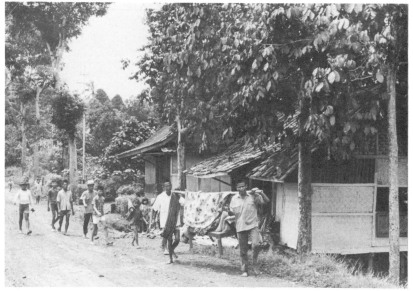

WHO Photo: K. Frucht

Patient referral may be hampered by problems of transportation.

- overloading of the hospital with inappropriate self-referrals, or poorly-judged referrals;
- barriers of distance, transport, or payment;
- lack of confidence in health care at the health post/centre levels, leading to by-passing of those levels; and
- inadequate flow of information to and from the hospital.

Other problems were considered to be:

- inappropriate hospital use because of the lack of support and facilities in the community for people who find it difficult to live independently;
- lack of trust between the hospital and community-oriented services, often because of the absence of organizational and personal links;
- lack of a well-designed referral system with defined procedures, management support, and appropriate forms;
- lack of information (at each of the four primary health care levels) on the available facilities and capabilities of the local or regional health services;
- lack of logistic support;
- inadequate training or guidance at each level on referral criteria, and on which conditions should be referred to particular levels of the system; and
- the off-loading of patients by community services to the hospital because they are overburdened or because health workers lack adequate knowledge or training.

Overcoming the problems: approaches to solutions

With so many pitfalls along the way it might seem surprising that any nation has managed to install a reasonably successful system of referral, whether in the specific sphere of individual patient care or in the more nebulous area of what the Expert Committee calls "referral of administrative and management problems". Nevertheless, some countries obviously do succeed to a greater or lesser extent and the Expert Committee report (7) quotes a number of the lessons to be learned from these.

Practical experience from a number of countries that have developed successful referral systems indicates the general importance of:

– recognizing that the whole referral system, from family to health posts/centres and the first referral level hospital, should be viewed as an integral part of the district health system;
– developing the referral system in consultation with potential users (providers and consumers), testing it, and providing mechanisms for review and the introduction of refinements until the system is working well;
– ensuring that contacts between hospitals and health centres are frequent and close, so that staff know and have confidence in one another; and
– avoiding over-rigid procedures so that various options for referral exist.

(i) *Patient referral.* Turning more specifically to patient referral, experience suggests the importance of:

– ensuring that the hospital concentrates on its role as a referral centre for a district, and does not do work that can equally well be done by community health centres (this may require the establishment of a 'health centre within the hospital', so that patients from the immediate neighbourhood do not use the hospital's referral resources as a preferred source of first-contact care);
– treating patients from health posts/centres as referred patients (i.e., not subject to additional delays or costs), and avoiding duplication of investigations;
– referring patients back as soon as possible to the source of referral, and with full information;
– introducing financial incentives/disincentives (for example, charging a fee to patients who have referred themselves to the hospital when they could and should have gone to a health post/centre);
– developing manuals of procedures and protocols for referrals, while still encouraging flexibility;
– making referral easy and convenient by having well-designed forms readily available, with some facts already completed by clerical staff so that the referring person only needs to fill in the parts of the form that relate to the patient's health; and
– considering local cultural requirements, especially in matters of privacy, such as who can examine women, and in what circumstances.

(ii) *Referral of administrative and management problems.* Within this very broad heading, the evidence available to the Expert Committee highlighted the importance of:

97

- enabling the hospital to provide logistic support to peripheral health care units;
- developing intersectoral collaboration to help overcome communication and transport barriers and other obstacles to progress;
- obtaining information on health care resources and capabilities in the area, and making it available to the community as well as to the providers of care so that everyone concerned knows who is likely to be the most appropriate person to help or advise them;
- developing appropriate training and supervisory mechanisms for community health workers and field staff, including traditional birth attendants and healers;
- ensuring that hospital staff play appropriate roles in educating community health workers and other staff based at health posts/centres, and in health promotion (but without ever being patronizing);
- recognizing the role of traditional medicine; and
- developing mechanisms for evaluating the main aspects of performance, including access to care, technical effectiveness and efficiency, acceptability, and outcome. This is an essential component of district health care management; the accent should be on quality assurance, not on measurement of performance for its own sake.

All this must make it patently obvious to the dispassionate critic that referral systems, whether for the sort of health care service we recommend or for any other, are easier to discuss than implement—a conclusion supported by the Expert Committee:

Referral systems are easy to design but extremely difficult to put into practice. The effectiveness of a referral system will depend on the patients' confidence in the different levels of the health system; the trust they have in the personnel; the effectiveness of the information system; the ease or difficulty of transport and the time spent travelling; the costs of care at different levels; and so on. Ineffective referral that by-passes the peripheral units to reach the hospital, or returns a patient to the periphery without useful information, actually sabotages the effectiveness of all parts of the system, the hospital no less than the others.

Overcoming the problems: some practical examples

If a study of health referral systems does nothing else, it serves to remind anyone who undertakes it that cooperative human activity of any kind is only possible where there is good communication between those involved. Goodwill, it is true, can help to make even the worst organization operable, but if reasonable communication is lacking any cooperative venture will fail.

In parts of India, for example, it seems that patient referral systems are poor because, *inter alia*, patients going from a primary health service to hospital are given no proper referral slip, and feedback from the hospital to the referring point is rare. India hopes to remedy some of these defects as a result of a variety of actions taken during its seventh Five-Year Development Plan, which ends in 1989.

Other countries, as might be expected, are following different approaches to the improvement of communications and so of referral systems. Some, like Kuwait, are small enough to have set up a centralized information system based on regional centres, which is designed to give every individual citizen a health care number and so facilitate their care and treatment wherever and whenever it is given.

As might be expected, activities in other countries are more localized. In Kenya, as in a number of other countries where health care facilities are widely dispersed, the basic emphasis has been placed on improving access to the health posts, centres and hospitals. Where telephones, good roads, and reliable vehicles are available—as in the Nyeri district of Central Province—dependable referral systems can be implemented. Where they are not, such systems cannot be provided.

In Nepal, national planning aims to produce a referral system that will link local communities to the central hospitals via four intermediate levels—health posts and district, zonal and regional hospitals. Meanwhile, the Patan Hospital operates a system locally which, although far from perfect, works well enough in practice. It involves the use of a two-sided, return referral slip, sent with the patient from the health post and returned there by mail from the hospital when the consultation and treatment are completed and the patient returns to the care of the health post staff. The slip includes a portion for completion which allows insured patients to reclaim reimbursable costs, and a carbon copy of the whole form, sent from the health post to the hospital's Senior Public Health Nurse, provides a means of monitoring all referrals. District patients so referred receive preferential treatment in the hospital with no registration fee chargeable, separate registration arrangements available and the opportunity of more direct access to the doctor. Similar concessions are available in whole or part, to patients referred from other sources, but not, one assumes, to those who are self-referred.

Systems not unlike that in operation at the Patan Hospital exist in many countries, as do various arrangements for interaction between hospital and primary health care workers. Such interactions, whether for education, training, clinical, or even social purposes, are to be encouraged. Referral systems of all kinds can undoubtedly be enhanced by personal contacts.

Chapter 9. Gaining ground

In the preceding chapters we have proposed that the advent of the WHO health for all strategy could herald a change in health care provision throughout the world that will be nothing short of a revolution.

In this final chapter we sum up our views on the aims of the health care revolution, assess the extent to which those aims have been achieved so far; and hazard a guess at future progress. We do this in three sections: what has to be done; what has been done; and what remains to be done.

What has to be done

The objective of the health care revolution, in a nutshell, is the creation worldwide of a system based on primary health care, of which hospitals must form an integral part.

But of course there is more to it than that, and we believe that we can do no better than quote the views of Dr Halfdan Mahler, Director-General of WHO, as presented in the keynote address that he gave to the inaugural session of the Conference on the Role of Hospitals in Primary Health Care, sponsored jointly by the Aga Khan Foundation and WHO, in Karachi, Pakistan from 22 to 26 November 1981 (6).

We make no apology for quoting extensively from Dr Mahler's address in which he enumerates five aspects of the association between hospitals and primary health care essential to successful implementation of the health for all strategy.

First, he comments on why the achievement of better health care for everyone depends on the institution of good primary health care sevices.

Primary health care is the key to attaining health for all by the year 2000. It consists of essential health care based on practical, scientifically sound and socially acceptable methods and technology, made universally accessible to individuals and families in the community through their full participation and at a cost that the community and the country can afford to maintain at every stage of their development, in the spirit of self-reliance and self-determination. . . . primary health care must become the central function and main focus of a country's health system. . . . As health development extends well beyond the sphere of the health services and the roots of health lie largely outside the health sector, there is, in addition, a need for close cooperation among the different sectors of development. Intersectoral cooperation, just as active community participation, is therefore a basic characteristic of the primary health care approach.

This is vastly different from the health system in most countries, in which the hospital is the hub of the system towards which patients, cadres, equipment and funds flow. However, the hospital's role in a health system based on primary health care is no less important—I would even submit that it is more important.

Secondly, he speaks about the need for hospitals in the new integrated national health systems to support primary health care in a number of important ways.

In supporting primary health care, front-line hospitals will act as a focal point for referrals. Patients needing special facilities and expertise will be referred to them by the first-contact level and referred back to that same level when their state of health permits it. . . .

Another no less important responsibility is support to communities, and to health workers providing primary health care, with respect to all the health problems that they encounter. This support should take the form of providing guidance and advice, continuous technical backup and supervision, continuing education and adequate follow-up of patients released from hospital, and monitoring of agreed health programmes.

Front-line hospitals should also provide managerial support to the planning and organization of the health system in the district, and to the organization of primary health care by communities. . . .

Another facet of support is what is known as logistics. This includes the supply of drugs; transport; communication; basic equipment; spare parts; maintenance of equipment, vehicles and buildings; and like matters, to keep the peripheral health care units running.

Thirdly, he looks at ways in which the people in the community served by a front-line (or first-referral level) hospital, may be encouraged and enabled to promote their own better health.

> The front-line hospital should play a leadership role . . . encouraging community decision-making and control . . . in combating bad health habits and promoting good ones, and in achieving adequate health services, all in the spirit of self-reliance.

They should use their "great human and technical resources . . . to provide the public with properly validated information on health problems and on appropriate technology for solving them."

And if they wish to be involved, as they should, in such fields as "nutrition, population, environmental health or water supply, [they] will have to cooperate closely with a host of other development sectors, including agencies responsible for food production and rural development."

Fourthly, he considers the need for good basic and continuing education of health workers—a need that hospitals must help to meet with radical changes in their training and educational methods.

One fundamental change that must be accepted, for example, is the principle that the person with the *least* formal training able to do a job should be the one to do it.

Another is the move away from training based on the curative, highly technological, sophisticated and dehumanized style of care, that many hospitals currently provide, and towards the more practical, field-based, community-oriented, people-centred form of caring which is enshrined in the primary health care approach.

> In this 'teaching hospital without walls', the learners, the future health workers, will learn how to function in teams both in the hospital and outside it in the community. They will not only learn how to analyze community health situations, and serve, support, guide and educate communities and individuals in their fight for health, but will also become socially motivated to do so. This kind of hospital will provide the learners with real life experience in health development, in health promotion, in prevention and rehabilitation and not just in curative care. . . .
>
> [Continuing education of health workers] too has to change in character. It can no longer remain at the level of 'provision of information'. Continuing education of all workers concerned with health has to relate to their problems, which are the day-to-day problems of people . . .
>
> [It] should also serve the reorientation of existing health workers so that they can perform optimally in an integrated health system based on primary health care. Training in the relevant parts of the managerial process for health development should form an integral part of such education. . . .
>
> Our movement for health for all will stand or fall with the success or failure of our efforts to prepare the future generations of health development workers for community oriented team-work in the spirit of the primary health care approach.

And, fifthly, he reminds us that hospitals will have responsibilities to "become involved . . . in the kind of research that aims at discovering the most efficient and effective ways of applying appropriate health technology, whether through primary health care or by the supportive hospital system, and at finding behavioral alternatives to such technology."

By such means, Dr Mahler concludes, may hospitals "be converted into agents for the service of society instead of precincts for individual medical transactions between doctors and patients . . . [and] become one of the main flag bearers of the most daring yet most promising health movement in the history of humanity. . . "

What has been done

Manifestly, as Dr Mahler saw the world situation in 1981, there was much to be done if the concept of health for all were to have any hope of becoming reality by the year 2000. Seven years later the position is not so very different, although obviously considerable progress has been made in the interim as witness the attention that has been given to the programme of health for all in every one of the six WHO Regions, and in every country of the world.

Actual measurement of the progress is difficult but it is clear that progress will have varied and will continue to vary widely from country to country, and especially across the great divide that separates the wealthier from the poorer countries. For example, health for all must be much further away at present in many parts of Africa, Asia, and Latin America than it is, say, in Europe and North America.

Nevertheless much has been achieved in many parts of the world. The International Hospital Federation's Study of 1981–83, mentioned on page 61, gives considerable support to this contention, particularly as far as the developing countries are concerned, as do the reports from individual hospitals and from the Royal Tropical Institute of Amsterdam, the Aga Khan Foundation, and the Christian Medical Commission.

A further cause for some satisfaction can be found in Table 2, which is taken from the report of a WHO Expert Committee (19). The table illustrates the improvement that

Table 2. Some quantitative health manpower indicators

	Population per physician		Population per nurse	
	1960	1980	1960	1980
Low-income countries	12 222	5 785	7 217	4 668
China	8 330	1 920	4 020	1 890
Ethiopia	100 470	58 490	14 920	5 440
India	4 850	3 640	10 980	5 380
Nepal	73 800	30 060	—	33 420
Pakistan	5 400	3 480	16 960	5 820
Zaire	79 620	14 780	3 510	1 920
Lower-middle-income countries	28 870	7 751	4 925	2 261
Brazil	2 670	1 700	—	740
Côte d'Ivoire	29 190	21 040	2 920	1 590
Egypt	2 550	970	1 930	1 500
Guatemala	4 420	8 600	9 040	1 620
Indonesia	46 780	11 530	4 510	2 300
Nigeria	73 710	12 550	4 040	3 010

has taken place over the twenty years up to 1980 in the number of professional health workers available in low-income and lower-middle-income countries. It is concerned only with doctors and nurses but in each case the improvement has been significant, although far from adequate.

As the report says:

> There have been substantial increases in the number of health personnel over the past 20 years; for example, using physicians as a general indicator of manpower, there has been an improvement in the population-to-physician ratio in the low-income countries from 38 000 to 16 000 (the World Bank excludes India and China from these figures) and in the lower-middle-income countries from 28 000 to 8 000.

But the report adds:

> Despite such improvements, extensive problems of health manpower development remain.

Special mention must be made of China, which is a striking example of what can be achieved in the development of improved health services given the necessary commitment to the task on the part of government, authorities and the people themselves.

The following is an extract from the conclusions of the Report of an Inter-regional Seminar organized by WHO, entitled *Primary health care—the Chinese experience (20)*.

> Among the countries of the world, one in particular—namely China, where almost a quarter of the world's population lives—has strikingly demonstrated how "health for all" can be achieved. During the exploration by the seminar of the four selected issues, through field work, direct observation, and intensive talks with the relevant health workers, and also during the discussions between the senior health administrators and the ministers and presidential advisers, a fundamental question was always present: what factors have contributed to the current high level of primary health care in China? Besides the many conclusions reached in respect of each of the four specific issues explored, some general factors emerged as having made a significant contribution.
>
> 1. China has demonstrated a tremendous political commitment to the task of changing the quality of life of all its people and especially of the rural population. Health goals have been given very high priority. This political commitment permeates all levels of government and all social and mass organizatons ensuring sustained popular support.
> 2. The reorganization of the country's economic and social structure, and in particular the high level of decentralization, has permitted the integration of

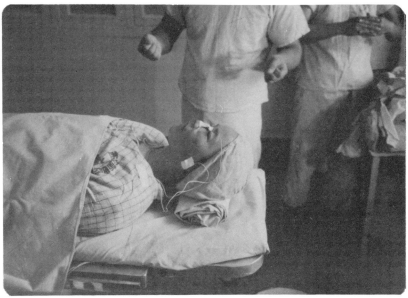

Photo: F. Siem Tjam

A contribution of traditional Chinese medicine: acupuncture anaesthesia.

the health sector with all aspects of economic and social development and has facilitated the people's involvement in the financing as well as the management of health care.

3. Concerted action in many sectors has contributed to raising the level of health of the people. Sufficient increase in income and its equitable distribution to permit minimally adequate shelter, clothing and, above all, essential food at affordable prices, the expansion of literacy and mass education (particularly primary education), the provision of public services such as water supplies and transport, the policies and programmes related to family planning, etc., have all contributed to this improvement in health status.

4. Perhaps the most important factor in the development of the health care system has been the participation of the people in the provision of health services, in the management of the system, and in mass campaigns. The people have contributed to the integration and better coordination of health programmes and to intersectoral collaboration at all levels.

5. Every step in the development of the Chinese health care system in the past—starting with mass mobilization for prevention, followed by the development of cooperative health centres, the emergence of the "barefoot doctor", the combined use of traditional Chinese medicine and western medicine, the development of the commune and brigade network with its cooperative medical insurance schemes and of the whole supportive health care network at higher levels, etc.—is a concrete and living expression of what constitutes appropriate technology.

107

Experience in China, therefore, shows all the principles of primary health care in operation. By studying it, a clearer idea can be gained of what primary health care is, and what it is not. For example, the participation of the people is not simply the contribution of community resources to a health system managed by professionals; nor is primary health care a matter of providing for community health workers with inadequate training, isolated from the rest of the health care system, unsupported and unremunerated by the people they serve. It is not an inferior system of health care, but rather a total system permitting all people to have access to the level of care they require at a cost that is within the means of the country and the individuals concerned. Finally, it is not a "programme" to be implemented in isolation either from other technical programmes in the health system or from other sectors outside the health system.

Action to improve primary health care also continues in developed countries spurred partly by the so-called "cost explosion" in health care—which has caused payers for services to look more critically at providers (especially hospitals) and hospitals to look more critically at themselves —and partly by a slowly rising tide of public opinion. "People", said Dr D. Tejada-de-Rivero, a former Assistant Director-General of WHO, "were realizing with increasing clarity that they were fast becoming passive objects under a medical care system far beyond their understanding and which they could neither participate in nor control" (2).

Finland and the United Kingdom have already been cited as examples of developed countries with a growing awareness of the need to develop the primary health care philosophy. They are not alone in this respect, and a number of countries are considering this approach as they seek solutions to the problems of deprived inner-city populations. This is reflected in the activities of the International Hospital Federation. Following on from the work that it did in the 1970s on health care in big cities (21), it has continued to organize annual workshops on health care planning in urban areas. At the tenth such gathering held in Stockholm in June 1986, the cities represented were Amsterdam, Copenhagen, Dublin, Lisbon, Nantes, Nottingham, Stockholm, and Thessaloniki.

However, activity is not confined to Europe. For example, a few years ago, the American Hospital Association and the University of Washington conducted a six-year study of hospital-sponsored primary care group practices in the United States of America; also the Australian Hospital Association has an annual awards scheme for outstanding

efforts by hospitals that involve themselves in primary
health care (2).

What remains to be done

One way of looking at the task that still confronts those
who pursue the goal of health for all by the year 2000 is
to think again of the differences between the 'haves' and
the 'have-nots' of the health care world.

It is self-evident that, however primary health care is
defined—as a level of care, a strategy for health for all, or
a philosophy for equity and social justice—the developed
countries have more of it than the developing ones. It
remains a fact that in the industrialized nations primary
health care workers are largely professional people—doctors,
nurses, social workers, health visitors, and trained
paramedical staff. In the poorer nations they are not.
Indeed, to quote Dr Tejada-de-Rivero again:

It is not unusual in developing countries to find between 40% and 60% of the
population without access to *any form* of permanent health care.

When discussing the improvement that took place between
1960 and 1980 in the number of professional health workers
available in poorer countries, we suggested that there was
reason for only limited satisfaction. Dr Tejada-de-Rivero's
statement makes clear our reason for so restrained a
congratulatory comment, as does a 1980 publication of the
King Edward's Hospital Fund for London (22).

Concerned with international comparisons of health needs
and services, the latter booklet looks, *inter alia*, at the
numbers of doctors and nurses available in thirteen
developed countries in the first half of the 1970s.

As regards doctors, the USSR headed the list at that time
with one for every 34 people, while England and Wales
brought up the rear with a ratio of 1:770. Corresponding
figures for nurses ranged from approximately 1:170 in
Sweden to 1:625 in Japan.

Just compare these data with those reproduced in Table 2
on page 105. The report from which these figures were taken
(19) goes on to say:

The shortage of certain categories of health worker remains a common problem in the developing world. In the least-developed countries there is 1 health worker per 2400 people compared with 1 per 100 people in the industrialized countries. Moreover, the unsatisfactory deployment of these health workers is such that the majority of them, often 80%, are working in and around urban areas where only about 20% of the population live. Few countries have a manpower distribution pattern that conforms to the real needs of the community, and health personnel often work within a health system that offers no career structure and few or no job incentives.

And as Sanders & Carver point out (4):

Of course not *all* parts of underdeveloped countries are underdeveloped. In fact the general pattern the world over is one of very uneven development, with grotesque inequalities, especially in the underdeveloped world. These inequalities are obvious to health workers who see and treat the *effects* of the inequalities.

In South Africa, for example, infant mortality rates are roughly six times as high for blacks and 'coloureds' as they are for whites. In other underdeveloped countries the poor and the rich are not distinguished by the colour of their skins and so there are no recorded infant mortality rates (or any other rates) for poor and rich, but rather rates for the population as a whole. . . .

In Africa and Asia there are even more striking differences in health between poor and rich. Infant mortality rates among élite groups in many parts of the underdeveloped world are similar to European rates—approximately 20 per 1000 live births—while the poorest people's infants die at a rate of up to 300 or even 400 for every 1000 born alive.

These are the sort of stark figures that must surely convince anyone with any pretension to a social conscience and sense of humanity that more must be done to redress this health imbalance. WHO has pointed the clear way forward, and there can be no doubt that we should all support, in every way we can, the strategy for health for all.

As we have already noted, much has been done since the Declaration of Alma-Ata in 1978. Primary health care activities have been encouraged and developed in homes, health posts, health centres, and communities, where emphasis is now being more firmly placed on self-reliance and on collaboration between a variety of organizations— governmental, nongovernmental and voluntary—concerned with the health and welfare of people.

These activities must obviously be continued and expanded but, equally importantly, so must the participation in primary health care of those centres of health care excellence, development, and privilege—the hospitals.

Indeed in its report, the WHO Expert Committee on the Role of Hospitals at the First Referral Level (7) issues a challenge to hospitals to examine their role as providers of first referral level services. It posed fourteen questions to be asked of hospitals. The questions, which are reproduced below, present key issues not usually recognized or faced up to by hospitals, and answering them calls for careful understanding of the technical, managerial, financial and social content of primary health care.

1. Does the hospital serve a specific population defined in terms of numbers, geographical boundaries, or other characteristics?
2. Does the hospital view its responsibilities as extending to the population outside its walls?
3. Does the hospital consider its role in primary health care to include participating in the characterization of the problems, resources, and needs of the population it serves?
4. Does the hospital consider it important to develop relations with all health agencies in the district, health practitioners of various types, community representatives, and authorities from other sectors in order to plan how the problems and needs of the population are to be dealt with?
5. Does the hospital participate in defining the prevalence and distribution of specific health problems (such as malnutrition, diarrhoeal diseases, complications of pregnancy, etc.), and help to plan who should be cared for outside the hospital and who should be hospitalized?
6. Does the hospital see its role as participating in the development and maintenance of an information system that would allow continuous assessment of the status of major problems affecting the population, monitoring of programmes directed at those problems, and evaluation of their effectiveness?
7. Does the hospital see its role as participating in health manpower development throughout the area it serves, including helping in recruitment, training, supervision, and evaluation of health workers?
8. Does the hospital consider itself to be responsible for providing logistic support (such as bulk purchasing and storage of supplies, maintenance of equipment, etc.) to local health services in the surrounding district?
9. With respect to referral of patients, does the hospital consider its role to include developing the criteria for the referral of patients from peripheral health workers, specifying the information that should accompany patients to and from the hospital, and training the various personnel to ensure the effectiveness of such referral arrangements?
10. In viewing the overall costs of primary health care for the district, does the hospital consider it reasonable that resources should be allocated across institutional boundaries?
11. Does the hospital consider the assessment of the quality of care to be an important approach to evaluating hospital functions, and would the hospital consider it appropriate to extend this approach to primary health care services in the surrounding district?
12. Does the hospital consider it necessary to make specific functional and organizational changes within the hospital in order to accommodate or facilitate its role in support of district-wide primary health care activities?

13. In evaluating its own performance, does the hospital consider its contributions to surrounding primary health care activities as important components of its programmes? How would the hospital assess its contributions? For example, would it use perinatal and infant mortality rates for the whole district or the extent of coverage of the populations as indicators of its performance?
14. Does the hospital consider it to be part of its role to join with community representatives and other interested parties in generating social and political support for the overall primary health care effort?

Let us, on this point, quote again from the address by Dr Lambo to the WHO Expert Committee:

Challenged by social needs and prodded by economic reality, many hospitals throughout the world are reacting in a variety of innovative ways. Some explore new interaction patterns while others initiate community health programmes or move to reorganize their structures to operate more in line with the primary health care approach . . .

It is clear that unless hospitals accept a partnership role and function in an integrated way with other services in the community, a fragmented local health system will persist. Hospitals should adjust to understand better the essential needs of the community they serve by developing an unprejudiced dialogue with all concerned with health, as equals engaged in the question for Health for All.

Governments, nongovernmental organizations and international organizations should promote this essential understanding so that past antagonisms may be converted into effective collaboration, thus ensuring the positive role hospitals must play in support of primary health care.

And assuming that "this essential understanding" is promoted, and that hospitals throughout the world are beginning to integrate with and support primary health care as they should, what is the health care revolution likely to have achieved by the beginning of the 21st century?

Once again it is fitting that the man who has striven so long and hard in support of this noble and humane campaign, should have the last word upon it. The quotation is from Dr Halfdan Mahler's paper (11), previously mentioned in Chapter 3.

In 1976 I chose to present to the Regional Committees the objective "Health for All by the Year 2000". The Thirtieth World Health Assembly in May 1977 took up this challenge by adopting a resolution urging "that the main social target of governments and WHO in the coming decades should be the attainment by all the citizens of the world by the year 2000 of a level of health that will permit them to lead a socially and economically productive life."

The purpose of this challenge is not to proclaim that all diseases and illnesses can be eliminated by the year 2000. Such a possibility is unimaginable; the vicissitudes of life are too great for anyone to dream of such a Utopia. No, this challenge is aimed at focusing world attention on the grave inequities that exist today and on the possibility of attaining an acceptable level of health, equitably distributed through the world in one generation's time. This is a realistic goal only if urgent action is initiated now. Primary health care is a viable alternative toward bringing about this objective. That we have made such little progress between 1937 and now should not be taken as evidence of the impossibility of the task. This heritage hangs heavily upon us. But I believe that this generation is up to the task of making the decisions necessary to correct this injustice.

If each individual country has the political courage both to reorient its internal health priorities according to their social relevance for the total national population and, simultaneously, to espouse the cause of international solidarity for global health promotion, then I have not the slightest doubt that we shall reach this goal before the year 2000.

References

1. *Alma-Ata 1978: Primary health care.* Geneva, World Health Organization, 1978 ("Health for All" Series, No. 1).
2. MACAGBA, R. *Hospitals and primary health care.* London, International Hospital Federation, 1985.
3. Organizational study on methods of promoting the development of basic health services. *Official Records of the World Health Organization,* No. 206, Annex 11, 1973.
4. SANDERS, D. & CARVER, R. *The struggle for health.* London, Macmillan Education Ltd, 1985.
5. MAHLER, H. Health—a demystification of medical technology. *Lancet,* **2**: 829–833 (1975).
6. *The role of hospitals in primary health care: a report of a conference sponsored by the Aga Khan Foundation and the World Health Organization, 22–26 November 1981, Karachi, Pakistan.* Geneva, Aga Khan Foundation/WHO, 1981.
7. WHO Technical Report Series, No. 744, 1987 (*Hospitals and health for all:* report of a WHO Expert Committee on the Role of Hospitals at the First Referral Level).
8. ROBERTS, F. *The cost of health.* London, Turnstile Press, 1952.
9. MILLER, H. *Medicine and society.* London, Oxford University Press, 1973.
10. LEAGUE OF NATIONS HEALTH ORGANIZATION. *Intergovernmental Conference of Far Eastern Countries on Rural Hygiene.* Bandoeng, Java (now Bandung, Indonesia), 1937.
11. MAHLER, H. Promotion of primary health care in Member States of WHO. *Public health reports,* **93** (2): 107–113 (1978).
12. NEWELL, K. W., ed. *Health by the people.* Geneva, World Health Organization, 1975.

Hospitals and the health care revolution

13. SANKARAN, B. The first referral level hospital. *World health*, September 1983, pp. 22–23.
14. DEPARTMENT OF HEALTH AND SOCIAL SECURITY. *Care in action*. London, Her Majesty's Stationery Office, 1982.
15. KING, D. *Down to earth planning*. London, International Hospital Federation Yearbook, 1987.
16. FARRANT, W. *Health for all in the inner city*. London, District Health Promotion Group, Paddington and North Kensington Health Authority, 1986.
17. MINISTRY OF SOCIAL AFFAIRS AND HEALTH. *Health care in Finland*. Helsinki, National Board of Health, 1986.
18. WILLIAMS, T. F. ET AL. The referral process in medical care and the university clinic's role. *Journal of medical education*, **36** (8):901 (1961).
19. WHO Technical Report Series, No. 717, 1985 (*Health manpower requirements for the achievement of health for all by the year 2000 through primary health care*: report of a WHO Expert Committee), pp. 10–11.
20. *Primary health care—the Chinese experience*. Report of an Inter-regional Seminar. Geneva, World Health Organization, 1983, pp. 73–74.
21. PAINE, L. H. W., ed. *Health care in big cities*. London, Croom Helm, 1978.
22. MAXWELL, R. *International comparison of health needs and services*. London, King's Fund Centre, 1980.